Getting Old Is A Hard Thing To Do

By Don Kirk

Getting Old

Is A Hard Thing To Do
By Don Kirk

The Golden Years?

Peace & Quiet?

San Antonio, Texas

Getting Old
Is A Hard Thing To Do
By Don Kirk

Published by
SWEETWATER STAGELINES™
An imprint of
THE OLD WEST COMPANY™
5118 Village Trail Drive
San Antonio, Texas 78218

Tradepaper (ISBN13): 979-8-88796-312-9
Printed and bound in the United States of America

Other books by Don Kirk available at
Lulu.com/spotlight/sweetwater
Amazon.com
barnes&noble.com

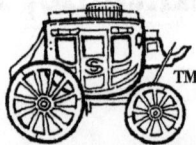

SWEETWATER STAGELINES™
SAN ANTONIO, TEXAS

Getting Old
IS A HARD THING TO DO
By Don Kirk

A few reviews, and commentary, to make you want to buy this book:

"The title is not inspiring. Who would buy this book? Especially the old dudes living it. Besides, getting old is EASY to do." —Tricia Carlson

"I read through it, but it was the very first article that put me to sleep." —Oliver Newton

"What an unoptimistic way to title it. How about 'The Golden Years.'" —Tommy Long

"It's not a fun thing to read. I guess the writer just wanted to get something off his chest." —Betty Molina

"You should name the book 'A Senior's Official Guide To Falling Apart!'" —Rich Kadiddlehopper

And on top of that, different fictional author's works were used to fill these pages.

Don Kirk

Getting Old Is A Hard Thing To Do
TABLE OF CONTENTS

Who Do I Have To Call?
—George Houston, 2022

A cloudy, gray-skied morning, everything's quiet except for a few irritated dogs. I'm walking mine. I feel like the sky looks: heavy, depressing, the world falling down on me. Where are the sunny bright mornings? I feel hopeless, why try to go on?

After 70, life becomes a chore: just going to bed and getting up, with multiple trips to the bathroom. And now today, what am I going to eat? Who do I need to call? How many years do I have left on this here planet?

Yes, life seems to be like weather that's marked by a covering of gray clouds, a little sunshine once in a while, but not very often.

I don't understand living. I walk the streets, the same streets—with my two dogs—looking at the environment. There is a certain unreality to the world around me: the cars, houses for "living" bumper to bumper across the landscape.

On this day, I'm walking through a public housing project and the weather is below freezing. There is no visible personage. No vehicles moving about, no birds perched on a telephone wire or flying about. No mysterious movements in the bushes. Getting old is like that: a dead dying atmosphere.

Trying to sleep is trying. It's work, it's stressful. I'm tired all the time. Everything is an effort, even getting out of bed…and falling into it.

Daytime life is boring, the same activities, same chores over and over, nothing new and exciting. Old folks sit in their one-hundred-year-old Chesterfield sofa watching TV all day long. The same programs over and over and over again, but they're not actually watching, just listening, if that, in a "devoid of life" state.

A boring life is boring, there's nothing to do; nothing you CAN do. You can't re-shingle a roof, crawl under the kitchen sink to fix a plumbing leak, or even change a light bulb on a ceiling fixture.

And my house is filled with, saturated with STUFF, but I call my things a hopeful name: "*Stupendously Tantalizing, Utterly Fantastic Findings.*" It's my S.T.U.F.F., good to someone someday. There is no longer room left to walk from room to room: lots of good collectibles, a narrow hallway to the rooms, but forget about going INTO a room. When getting old one has collected too much.

I've become dysfunctional, I can't concentrate; thoughts come and go faster than I can act on them.

I've walked into a VA hospital. Patients are standing about six feet apart and sitting thereabouts, all masked, mostly the elderly like myself, a bunch of gray-haired oldies. They're all quiet, no talking going on, a strange silence throughout the waiting room and hallways of this large hospital—something weird about it in this Covid-19 world; it's mechanized, inhuman.

I hear a bunch of musicians beating on drums and guitars and sucking on microphones with a large audience listening in the background. Where did it all come from? My brain is going, well breaking...

I'm looking at the world differently. It feels and looks different. Maybe like an abandoned house with flaking paint and grown up in weeds: silent, ignored.

The routine of it all: city busses passing that all look the same. Vehicles with open windows and loud music blaring from them. Barking dogs trapped behind chain-link fences all their precious lives. Acres of cars parked in front of gargantuan grocery stores.

Walking the neighborhood early in the morning, I see rows of houses and apartments with no sign of life. And there are no vehicles moving at all, a little peace and quiet.

I'm looking at the wild animals: the raccoons, possum, porcupines, birds, cats...and appreciate them more. Well, except for the felines lying on and under every nook and cranny.

I'm looking at the details of my environment more...plants, trees, cloud types in the sky...stratus, cirrus, cirrocumulus...

My memory continues to falter. I try to write down things, but by the time I've gotten a pencil and paper, I've forgotten what I wanted to write down!

"If at first you don't succeed, get someone else to do it." An old age rewrite of a proverb.

I see rows of housing; human beings are just honeybees in a hive, but without wings they use big heavy, expensive automobiles to move about.

I look at the national news media and see a lot of commercials broken up infrequently by news commentary with no actual unbiased reporting. People seem different, all older. My long-time friends are mysteriously grizzled, I don't recognize them!

Looking at politicians on television, I see them not as before, not legitimate, not trustworthy. And all of government, none of it working for the people…and they're demanding more and more money in taxes, and for what?

A homeless person with backpack was sitting curled up outside a nearby convenience store. He looked up from "his sleep," stood up, and asked me for money. I gave him a five-dollar bill and went inside. A few minutes later, he came into the store and bought two packs of cigarettes and several lottery tickets. There is something wrong here.

The Cliff Dwelling
—Bubba Bosley, 2021

I was with a friend exploring some, no many, amazing rooms carved into tall canyon walls at *Bandelier National Monument* in New Mexico; a cliff dwelling that housed human life over 11,000 years ago. It was a place I had been to many years earlier and now the interior seemed to have gotten much larger and absolutely full of "things" to look at as one makes his way through the maze of rooms: clay pots, cooking utensils, woven rugs, coat hangers (apparently from the ancient peoples), and even Indian arrows and headdresses from the more recent inhabitants…no, mostly were not originals, just nice reproductions covering the walls for us tourists to look at. The dwelling was like some kind of underground cave with excavated tunnels running off in every direction. It was built many hundreds, no thousands of years ago, dug out of the canyon walls, the interior sandstone a dark orange in color, meandering about, many rooms carved out of the canyon walls. Openings in every direction, no doors per se running from room to room. But now I needed to find a bath-room—us old folks need that often—so I told my friend I'd go find a John, and he should stay and wait for me here in this "room." I headed out looking, no wandering, through the various openings and rooms. Lots of things on display: lanterns, clocks, hand-made gizmos, very old books—walls covered solidly with them. I guess some were available for sale, just reproductions. I kept looking, and looking, and looking, no potty yet. I gotta go! I think I now had been looking what seemed like an hour! Finally, I asked an attractive-looking young lady for directions to the nearest toilet. She said I should use the GPS on my phone. Phone? GPS? I don't have a cell phone!

"Your *Global Positioning System* will get you to the restroom."

"In here?"

"Sure."

"Can I use yours? Will it show me where to go?"

The lady pulled her mobile phone from her pants pocket and slid her finger across the screen to the left and then right, up, and then down. "You can go that way, two rooms forward, turn right, up the ramp, walk left ten yards, small room to the right, through an opening to the East…"

I peed in my pants.

"How do I find my way back to that room with my friend?" I asked.

"Can you tell me where he is?"

"Are you kidding me?"

"No, the GPS will…"

I said thanks and walked off. I had no idea where to go. Room after room after room tied together with only small openings, not doors, none labeled and no blaring sunlight to give me a sense of direction. And when, and if I make it back outside, how would I find my car in the acres of H.E.B.-like parking lots? A nightmare in its own right, I, I…I woke up.

Getting Old
An Introduction
—Stew Longfellow, 2022

Getting old. It's a boring world, dreams merging with reality. The sameness of it all...day in and day out, nothing new and exciting, but now, on this day, do I want something exciting? Hell no, I want peace and quiet, to be left alone.

Basic bodily functions like urinating, bathing, trimming toenails, eating...all become necessary survival skills that require the utmost effort. Getting old.

I even have extreme mood changes on occasion: anger and irritability, anxiety and fear. And sometimes I have unending diarrhea and feelings of fatigue. And an ear infection, sinus congestion, runny nose...oh, it's just a cold. Skin infections, fragile fingernails, thin, easily ripped open skin...what ta hell? Getting old.

Tying on a pair of shoes with shoe laces wrapped all about, threaded in and out of little metal holes, such a time consumer, me all bent over, straining my back, I long ago had to switch to shoes with *Velcro* instead of laces. So much easier to put on, so that makes them harder to find in the shoe stores. Getting old.

I have a second new computer and it's causing nothing but more problems. With them damn frickin' passwords for one, no longer working in some cases. Websites don't know which computer is actually legitimate. Getting old.

I'm aging with my friends and neighbors and family dying all around me. I walk the streets daily for about three miles only to pass the houses of people I knew that are no longer breathing on this planet. Some of the meagerly furnished houses still have a spouse left, living alone...living with maybe a single cat to talk to, and family members rarely showing up. Getting old.

I even look, and listen to, old music differently. My past reminded by, "*Lay, Lady, Lay*" by Bob Dylan and "*Stairway to Heaven*" by Led Zeppelin. And then there is the *101 Strings Orchestra* playing "*Lawrence of Arabia*" and "*The Sound of Music.*" And it's not the words, the tune dissolves into my very being. Ageless music makes me feel old! Go figure. All my life now feels in the past. No present life. What will happen to the CD's of music I'm listening to now? What will happen to all that I've made and collected? Sitting at my computer, a female voice reminds me what time it is: "It's ten o'clock." I guess the computer even wants me to feel older, having to tell me what time it is. And I find myself talking to myself a lot. So what is that all about? Is it boredom, loneliness? Or just, ha, ha, two brains in one body talking to each other! But, *"Theme From The Magnificent Seven"* is still uplifting and hopeful. Getting old. (P.S. The greatest western film ever made was *"The Searchers"* starring John Wayne and directed by John Ford.)

Artificiality. An interstate highway fogged in, thick, near zero visibility, and billions of vehicles going somewhere every day. What kind of world is this? Everyone coming and going to work, day in and day out, year after year, a never ending nightmare, I'm ready to wake up. Getting old.

The clocks are ticking throughout the house. I hear them all in my head. They compete with the ringing in my ears. It's 5:00am and still quite dark—the room is my head; I'm IN my brain. It's doing nothing productive, just biding time, waiting to die.

Getting old.

GETTING OLD TWO
—Stew Longfellow's Brother

I'm tired of living. I'm tired of getting up every day. I'm tired of eating, and these routine activities lead to nowhere. I'm tired of listening to commercials, all the time, everywhere on everything. I'm tired of chores popping up that have to get done, or else. I'm tired of the phone ringing all the time—Robocalls. My computer, inundated with unsolicited email, the only way to communicate. Electronics: wouldn't it be nice if we suddenly had no electricity on this here planet! I just hope I have a few matches and a good pocketknife. But at least the human population would come to realize what in our life is really important.

I'm concerned at what will happen to all my life's work: the books I've written, artwork, photography, and museum collections that will all be sold off in an estate sale for a fraction of their worth. Committing suicide becomes more of a solution to my sadness, and so easy to accomplish. So, was life worth living in the first place? Are we just another of this planet's creatures trying to survive for a few years to reproduce and keep the species going?

From time to time my blood pressure jumps without apparent purpose. Stress? Yes, I'm stressed out by stuff, my things. I "live" in a warehouse. You'd have to see it to believe it: stacks to the ceiling of white file boxes with pathways between them, just twelve-inches wide requiring the moving of my body carefully sideways.

People driving while on their cell phones—"distracted driving" they call it. Cell phone use is completely out of control: 3,000 people died in 2018 talking on their phone while driving!

I see acres, miles and miles, of bumper-to-bumper racing automobiles; people trying to get somewhere; a scary reality in big, fast-growing cities like Houston and Dallas...and San Antonio.

Superstores like *Walmart* (and *Amazon*) are replacing the Mom and Pops. The profits go to the few, and billions of products come from China. Sounds like a democrat talking, no, just reality.

And I'm tired of doctors who give you these five-minute annual physicals! Their only info used to judge your health are the results of a blood draw.

Why should I be worried about any of this, I'll be dead soon.

Hang on, dear reader, there's much more about getting old. And not all is so distressing...or is it?

Getting Old
Just The Facts
—Audry Earp

That is all, jut the facts, there is nothing more:

I thought growing older would take longer.

I sometimes wonder what happened to the people who have asked me for directions.

When I can't remember the name of someone I know, to get their attention, I just say: "Want a beer?" and he'll turn around.

I don't do drugs and I don't drink. I can get the same effect by standing up too fast.

All right, I have an idea. Where's a note card so I can write it down? And here now, a pencil to write with. Oh wait, now I've forgotten the idea.

I've finally reached the wonder years, I wonder where my car is parked, I wonder where I left my phone, I wonder where my glasses are, and I often wonder what day it is.

The Story Of Getting Old
—Jeff Betters, 2018

Sorry, no story yet, but to remember things I make notes on notecards, but then I usually lose track of the cards. Here are the few I didn't:

Sidney and Joe are sitting at the *IHop* breakfast diner dragging their meals around with their forks as they converse about their love of getting old:

"I don't like this getting old, crap. That's the bottom line. My body and the world around gets me upset so easily," declared Sidney.

Joe, looking out the dinner window adds, "Heavy, dark gray, overcast skies seem to symbolize my feelings: depressing thoughts of life coming to an end."

"Yeah, sleeping is a chore. With insomnia and an enlarged prostate I can fall asleep for almost an hour—well, sometimes—and then I'm up to the bathroom..."

"You got that right," replied Joe, I too have to make frequent trips to the bathroom, day and night, so that means I have to stay close to one."

"As soon as I enter *H.E.B.* or a shopping mall, I look for the can."

Sidney takes a drink of his coffee. "I find myself talking to others of my age about our old age problems, and they all seem to have the same complaints and concerns."

Joe nods in agreement, "I find that I desire peace and quiet, no damn phone calls, no seeing of people, no going anywhere. I don't even have much desire to talk to my long-time friends."

"I think of nursing home living, how horrible that must be AND how costly it is."

"Me, I look at the sheer, monstrous sizes of places of business like *H.E.B.* and *Walmart.* What happened to the little corner store?"

"Well now, you've got the service station with a lot more than just gas."

"Television is now mostly commercials, yeah, one third of every hour; and they do a great job of destroying the pacing of the show."

"I can't watch television anymore," noted Sidney.

Joe reached for his scruffy beard, "I see more and more old folks growing beards, the white ones. In my case, it's just because I lost track of my razor."

"I believe that. Me, I can't seem to get anything done; very little progress is made on the different chores. You see, my list of things that need to get done gets longer and longer every day."

"The now complicated complexity of electronic devices, how can anyone operate these things? Vehicles, mobile phones, computers, light fixtures. I'm keeping my 1969 stick-shift Volkswagon beetle. And then there are passwords—for everything—that have to be so complicated to work. The computer. I remember when I typed holes in yellow IBM punch cards to input lines of code so I could program a gargantuan room-filling monster."

"Punch cards?"

"And I find myself stressed out about so many things like where is my 'retirement' money coming from since I don't have any retirement money; I just worked freelance."

Sidney took a drink from his orange-juice glass, "I can't answer my phone ringing without getting numerous Robocalls. Of course, frequently irritating, suddenly disturbing rings, so I plan to cancel my phone service. I will save money that way too. And the numerous letters and emails that look official, I just won't reply to any of them. From now on I'll have to communicate by postcard, my first one to everyone: 'I'm sending this postcard because my computer was successfully hacked and I lost all my email addresses and the phone advertising, hell, I'm cancelling my telephone number after 40 years. It was nice knowing you guys.' and you, Joe Dangford, this could be our last get together."

Getting Old
Are You Depressed?
—Terry Talbert, 2019

I see the beauty in a fighter's jet trail lit by early sunlight against a massive blue sky as it stretches almost horizon to horizon. A few high stratocumulus clouds are being moved south by a cold north wind and dark storm clouds are slowly moving in. I see symbolism in all that: life slowly changing for the worst. Anything could happen. I see life—my world—in a different light: thick, horizon-to-horizon, dull and boring, clouds.

A heavy, gray, depressing cloud bank sits neverendingly overhead, no sunlight for days; something imprisoning about it all. I'm living in a cardboard box…that hasn't been opened in a long time.

I feel like I'm stepping into the past when I drive to a part of town I haven't been to in years. It feels like I'm in another world… and I get lost easily, especially if the day is cloudy and there is no sun to give me a sense of direction. I easily get turned around… and lost.

My head is messed up, I can't think straight. I feel bad all the time; I don't know what is going on, help me here! I feel completely dysfunctional, useless, don't feel like doing anything, it's just this weird sickness I don't understand. I'm sick all the time.

And the boredom of routine. I could not do a job that required the same activity day in and day out over and over and over again, like the driving of a truck that picks up big brown 96-gallon trash cans all day long—or a meter reader reading water meters all day.

I look at all my long-time friends and they are all looking old! That's very scary because that means I must also be getting old. I'll have to take down my bathroom sink mirror so I won't have to look at my horribly, aging self.

I seem to have lost interest in anything and everything, as if I have run out of steam, don't care about finishing anything anymore. All those projects I had yet wanted to do, well, now I don't give a Flying Fitzgerald.

I've been a warehouse manager of antiques and miscellaneous collections and now I'm going through a life stage where I'm wandering what these seventy-one years have been about. All I'm leaving behind is a lot of frickin' junk, as valuable as it might be. Is a big garage sale the way to end a life, leaving behind what little you accomplished on planet earth? I should change my name to "Big Garage Sale" for what I accomplished. "Hey, Big, how you doing? Found anything cool lately at the flea market?"

With my memory getting worse, I try to take notes to remind me as to what I need to do; the trouble is, I can't ever remember where I left the notes. Yes, even if I put notes in my billfold to keep them close, I then forget they are there.

And I can't keep track of the medication I'm supposed to be taking for the illnesses I "might" have. Did I take this morning's? Did I take yesterday's? Sometimes I can't even tell you what day of the week it is. I can't even remember what I did the day before. Sometimes a friend tells me something we did together and I have no effin memory of it!

My ears are ringing louder and louder, my memory clearly getting worse. And it's only days before federal income taxes are due and I can't, dat burn it, remember if I even did them! No memory of it. In a panic, I start looking on my computer and through paper files. It turns out I had indeed completely finished that task, definitely a relief...except for the fact that I had absolutely NO memory of that piece of work.

The *PowerBall* lottery is ready to pay a winner one billion dollars! All that money, and more, paid by the poorest citizens of America. Look at how much of their hard-earned money they are throwing away. And are they using these new free government payments to have lots of kids?

Television, how primitive is that? I look at these current and old TV programs much more objectively and think of all the people sitting there staring at a flickering screen that's showing thousands of old reruns.

I look at people differently now. They are just another planetary creature moving around in some kind of four-wheeled vehicle and roaming around with metal baskets in big grocery stores. We are streets full of ants in a massive anthill: many hundreds of postmen delivering mail, numerous Fedex and UPS trucks delivering online purchases, and walls and walls of eighteen wheelers racing somewhere. Almost everyone is living next to railroads and expressways in the big cities, and acres and acres of automobiles are parked along the streets, and speeding down clogged-up highways. Thousands upon thousands of vehicles, bumper to bumper every day. And speeding-fast gambling with people's lives. At night, hell on earth: vehicles with glaring headlights and braking red taillights. Everyone trying to get somewhere at the same time…ahead of everyone else, in a nonsensical hurry.

After seeing miles and miles of housing in every direction, over hill and over dale, like the massive Indian pueblos of New Mexico, and looking at the acres and acres of today's multi-storied apartments, I don't see much difference.

I see green and red *Dempster Dumpsters* surrounded with piles and piles of worn-out furniture pieces—life ends in piles and piles of junk. No, I'm not depressed, not me.

All these old farts in congress—with ugly suits and ties—making decisions for us? They've been in office it seems forever, a career doing what? Making lots of money and great deals for themselves. We certainly need a revision of the system. Like term limits. Two terms maximum.

All these electronics in a digital world that's gotten all too complicated. Everyone inter-connected by a few finger-typed *Twitter* truncated "sentences"—just a few words used to express themselves. *Over The Air Television*, how mundane is that? And all those damn commercials. One has to be awfully bored to sit there waiting for the story to continue after those numerous howling ads. Play poker or *Scrabble*, dress your dog. OTAT will surly be completely eliminated, replaced by commercial-less *Nexflix*, and *Amazon*.

When I walk the streets with my dogs I pass, over and over, the houses where people I used to know once lived, and are now dead and buried. And homes where only one person, a former husband or wife, who lives alone now, eking out a survival; emptiness not just in the house but in the body. IN the body. And then that person also eventually dies and the house goes up for sale. So very sad. Just a temporary time on this planet. Are these humans?

A truck deliveryman dropping off what have you. It's got to be a lonely life working by yourself. Seeing his fellow workers only in the morning when loading up his truck. And then saying "see you tomorrow" when he returns to the station.

At my elderly age I'm more aware of everything. I look at every detail much more closely. And I talk to myself over and over and over again. So what gives? Is this depression?

I look at television advertising and the national news as so much crap. There's a constant push to buy, buy, buy. They want you to spend every penny you've made, and then some. And the news is just biased commentary, no investigative reporters on staff. The public and the national news networks get their news from *Facebook* and *Twitter*. Yes, really, plenty of documented cases.

I get up in the morning feeling totally tired...and it stays that way all day. I feel like I haven't slept in a week. What's going on here? Depression?

With the *Daylight Savings Time* change in November, the light is different for this time of the year. Another sense of the artificiality of it all. What is real? A creative sunrise, with the world only partially lit, adds to the mystery. The moon is still high in the sky and its already midmorning! Something is out of kilter. I'm thinking of those friends that have died before their time. Life is so out of wack. Heavy fog this early morning, the world seems so surreal, like a painting, ocean waves but no sound to go with it...

I get sudden flashbacks triggered by a smell, and then a sick feeling comes with it. I'm sitting in front of my computer, or at the kitchen sink, wide-awake, and suddenly I get an image of a past event! It only lasts a second or two and then I can't recall what it was. A real mystery, these brain neuron memory cells doing something, but what?

I'm sick in a strange way. The world feels somehow different. Not the same as I've been used to. My long-time friends look and sound old! There's sometimes a feeling from the past, but for only a second, while working, walking the dog, watching a TV program. The image and then a sickness! Yeah, I'm sick all the time, but other than that I'm fine.

I look up at a night sky to see a moon partially obscured by fog. I look at my carpentry and maintenance tools, at my house, the street, the cars, it's just not the same.

Suddenly, the sun breaks through some clouds on the horizon and the clouds turn deep dark orange. It's an amazing sight that never gets old to watch. Dark orange reflected off dark gray clouds, not quite real, more like a video game.

Life is amazingingly wonderful. We're only here for a short time with all these many creatures on this planet trying their best to survive. And evolving over millions of years. We humans came from chimpanzees. Appreciate that. If I drive carefully, stay off the freeways, and win that million-dollar Lottery Ticket...there's still hope.

—notes from a pocket voice recorder, Feb, 2019.

A quote from Barney Miller:
"Fish, why you feelin' so bad?"
"It's either a paranoid depression or
something I ate for breakfast."
"What did you eat for breakfast?"
"I didn't eat breakfast."

GETTING OLD
QUOTATIONS
From Some Well Knowns

Some random 'Getting Old" quotes:

"We're just like an old jalopy: a clunker where one part breaks down and then another, and we try to fix and replace what we can, but time is not on our sides." —Don Kirk

"If these will be my golden years, I don't want to be gold. I'll be nickle, or copper, or silver, or something else." —Lillie Fairfield

"I was thinking about how people seem to read the bible a lot more as they get older, and then it dawned on me—they're cramming for the final exam." —George Carlin

"Besides,' continued Julian, 'you can slam down a phone like that. You can't slam down a mobile. Imagine, a whole generation who'll never know the joy of slamming down a phone." —Clare Pooley

"You know you're getting old when you stoop to tie your shoelaces and wonder what else you could do while you're down there." —George Burns

"I'm at an age when my back goes out more than I do." —Phyllis Diller

"By the time you're 80 years old you've learned everything. You only have to remember it." —Bill Vaughan

"If you're not getting older, you're dead." —Tom Petty

"I don't feel old. I don't feel anything until noon. Then it's time for my nap." —Bob Hope

"Laughter is timeless. Imagination has no age. And dreams are forever." —Walt Disney

Man Without A Body
-Larry DoLittle, 2003

A former surgeon, Dr. Albert Johnson, who had always worried what would happen to his career if he injured or lost his hands, now finds himself with no legs, no arms, and no body! What remained was just his head—a skull and brain wrapped in muscle tissue, it setting inert on a wooden sculpted pedestal that had been used for a potted plant. The Head smiled sickly with a painful, crooked grin.

The man without a body had no full-time help, a nurse three times a week and a neighbor that would come over to visit him every few days. The neighbor, concerned about the doctor's eternally depressed state, would sit and talk to him from time to time.

A movie star's face when young, he was dignified, handsome and mature, but the age lines were beginning to reflect and even eclipse his actual age. There were crevasses around his mouth and eyes caused by his loneliness and lack of facial-muscle exercise. On his middle-aged head were graying, short stubbles of hair that would be trimmed from time to time. He had no friends to smile or laugh with; no longer any consulting with grateful patients after a successful surgery, and no colleagues that made any effort to come by and visit him.

Dr. Johnson was braced there upright on his neck with eight clear plastic tubes emanating from his neck, going through a hole in the pedestal top, and running to a large re-circulating heart pump housed in stainless steel and sitting on casters so that his head could be moved around to some degree, maybe to provide him with a different view on occasion, though no one had moved him since being placed in his home and he couldn't move himself.

The doctor's home was perched on the cliff of an Oregon Pacific Coast coastline—a house of modest size designed by an award-winning architect—with stairs winding in every direction to multiple levels, to rooms that the surgeon knew he would never be able to return to. The house was designed and engineered so well that it looked like it belonged, that it merged successfully with nature like moss on ocean-side rocks.

The surgeon thought, if I could just get out through that sliding glass door—the door that revealed a beautiful view of the ocean, the door that opened to a rocky cliff and wild surf far down below—if I could just roll out the door and fall into that surf, crashing against the granite rock, if only...but sadly I have no method of mobility. I will have to get someone to do it for me. I must convince my help to do something as simple as throwing a 22-ounce basketball over the railing, something a dog could do—though the human head is a bit heavier, weighting in at about ten pounds. It could be done by even the smallest of adults—someone with two hands and a pair of legs...

You see, the doctor had no desire to continue his morbid life.

When his head was first severed, he remembered his body dancing for a moment like a headless chicken, bright red arterial blood spurting from his neck, splattering on the white popcorn ceiling. He couldn't remember where his head had flopped to; he had only hoped there would be a nice wicker basket with a pillow.

His life was a life of the mind, a brain always thinking, though he had no control over it, like those sleepless nights he had before the accident. A wandering mind, totally out of control, keeping him awake when he needed to get a sound sleep before a four a.m. surgical procedure. Now, in a half-awake dream state, he imagined he still had all of his appendages and his surgical practice. He could see his nimble hands as he pulled on his surgical gloves. He could see the nurses standing around him, though sometimes they would pull down their surgical masks in unison and grin at him.

But he did have one welcome consolation: he had a nice trusting beagle, twenty-five pounds, short legs, large floppy ears with a brown, white, and black coat. She wasn't the smartest dog in the world, but she would come to lick the doctor's face every time he had a facial itch. It was the one sensation he could control. You see, he would use a hard-wired brain sensor to activate his home computer to yell out "Here, Lucy!" and the dog would quickly oblige. Lucy would lay quietly beside him, always ready and waiting for his command to lick.

The accident. The doctor knew what was going to happen just before it did. The realization just as it happens that you have made a mistake and now can't take it back, like climbing a ladder you knew was not sitting quite level. You can't do it over, no Time Machine to repeat the past. Yes, the doctor survived the ordeal by sheer circumstances beyond his control, something contrary to all of his training: to be in control at all times. He was in the operating room—the perfect place to have a life threatening injury: nurses, doctors, and masked technicians ready to jump into the *Code Red* emergency mode—as a large sliver of glass seriously severed his neck. The heavy overhead surgical light broke from its moorings, falling straight for him. He looked up, watching his life pass before his eyes. He had pulled the fixture too hard, trying to get it closer to his work, and he knew it, but too late. The light's lens shattering on him.

He was unconscious for over a minute, but in that time, the bleeding was arrested and a temporary blood pump of sorts was attached to the carotids and jugulars emanating from his neck. The mechanical heart, delivered to his home with him, was able to provide the necessary nutrients and oxygen to his brain cells and the muscle tissue of his head. It weighted a whole lot more than his former eight-ounce heart. Without his body, it took some time for his brain to adjust to the absence of information from the brain stem. The doctor understood that the nervous system had to have been severely traumatized, but here he was, still alive... as it were.

Dr. Johnson's neighbor, who lived about three miles way down off the hilltop, on this day, came to pay "The Head" a visit:

"How are you doing, Doc?"

The doctor looked toward him and tried to crack his crooked, painful-looking grin.

"Good, good. I'll check your pump. I guess they still don't make heart pumps quite like the real thing."

"Oxygen-rich blood to the cerebellum," the doctor replied to himself, but he was quite stressed out, and it showed with blood flowing faster through his supply tubes and flushing his face beet red. How could he tell his neighbor what he really wanted from him: to roll his Godforsaken head out the sliding glass door and into the ocean. The doc could answer "yes" or "no" questions by rolling his eyes, but he knew his neighbor had no idea what to ask. "How are you doing, Doctor?" was usually as far as it went. Instead of asking, "Is the heating thermostat to your liking, is the light level okay for you, should I close the curtains, can I get you some fresh air?" he should be straight with me and ask, "Do you want to die?" The doctor so wanted to reply to that question, turning his eyes upward to mean, "yes, you're damn straight I want to die!"

"Your pump looks fine. The nurse said you'll be getting some new blood next week."

Maybe it would be from a pig with the Ebola virus, the doctor thought. He had also hoped that a lightening storm would bring down the power lines. The electric current would stop flowing and his blood would quickly dry up. Unfortunately, even if the power to the house failed, there was a gas-operated backup generator.

"Can I set up your Book Page Flipper and get you a good detective novel to read? The latest surgical procedures?" he would ask me. You've got to be kidding!

The doctor lowered his eyeballs and the sides of his mouth drooped. He couldn't even tell his nice neighbor what he'd like to read. The neighbor would just grab something off the bookshelf—usually medical manuals he would never again have a use for. But the doctor couldn't read the books anyway; the text now appeared slightly out of focus; he was now in need of eyeglasses. He could just imagine his lone head sitting on a high stool in an optometrists' office as they tried to give him an eye exam for a prescription. Quite a sight. And would they give him one pair of glasses for reading and another for distance? He sure couldn't switch the two himself. And he sure couldn't use bifocals; that would require the moving of his head up and down! Just for a brief moment there was an internal momentary laugh. The sad helplessness of it all was actually funny.

"No, then how about the television? I can set it to your favorite channel," added the neighbor.

The doctor rolled his eye sideways—old television shows, or the CNN news all damn day long! No, thank you.

If only he'd ask me the right questions. Then maybe, just maybe, I could convince the neighbor to accidently kick the pump's electrical extension cord from its wall socket...if only...just a little kick, that's all I need.

The computer voice went off, "Here, Lucy!"

The neighbor jumped back in surprise as "Lucy," quickly jumped up from her sleeping repose. The hound climbed on a step and stood up on her hind legs to lick the doctor's face.

And the doctor didn't have to pay any insurance co-payments so they had no reason to shut off his pump. Even the house, this nice home overlooking the Pacific Ocean with it's wonderful sunsets almost every evening, was completely paid for, with property taxes and all utilities coming out of his estate—he was dead and not quite dead, an undetermined condition for who knows how long—in limbo for all of eternity? The mechanical heart would just be replaced when it wore out, but he—his head and brain—how long would that last? A mouth with a wilted tongue and useless set of teeth, a few more wrinkles on his face. He knew the folds and bulges of his brain looked like a large succulent meaty walnut and his face would eventually look much the same. His larynx—the voice box—was gone or crushed, but even so, it was part of the respiratory system so it couldn't function without the air pressure in the windpipe exhaled from the lungs; no lungs no voice. He thought, there will never be any way to communicate with the outside world. "Very literally taken, everything outside my head can no longer be interacted with—except maybe with my eyes. I can roll them, move them left or right, and close my eyelids. If only...The cliff was just out there, just beyond the glass door, just beyond the screen door and the deck's railing. My head could easily roll under the bottom rail and fall freely downward."

The doctor finally had a promising idea. If he could just teach Lucy a few "tricks," get her to follow a few basic commands. She was a very smart dog, descendent of two of the top ten smartest. The doctor would just need training treats and the dog would respond to the doctor's eye movements, left, right, up, down.

Lucy sat in front of the pedestal, looking up at the doctor. The doc looked to the left and then back to the center. He repeated this task many grueling times until the dog finally also looked to the left. When the dog did, he executed, with his mind, the computer to say "Here, Lucy" and the dog jumped up to lick his face. The doctor realized this could be a way to reward the dog for good behavior instead of using an edible treat. He repeated this whenever the dog was sitting before him looking curious and waiting for the next command. He did the to-the-left look until the dog did it on every occasion. Then he started in with the looking-right routine until Lucy caught on, and the learning curve became much faster.

He wanted the dog to jump, hitting his face with her front paws instead of the pedestal top. He used his upward eye movement as the command and rewarded Lucy every time she jumped a little higher. When the time was right, the doctor would do this again and again until she pushed him over. The doctor then came up with eye blinking as another sign to get the dog to do something. He could use one, two, or three eye blinks, and Lucy would be able to recognize their difference because of a dog's ability to distinguish detailed movements better than even a human can.

Now he wanted the dog to turn and go toward the sliding glass door so she would eventually drag The Head toward it. To train her to do this, he would blink twice and wait until the dog craned her neck to look outside after hearing an unusual sound like people talking on the beach or a seagull flying by. He had plenty of time to wait for the right moments, and would quickly reward her with "Here, Lucy," a pleasurable lick to the doctor's face. It worked, better than he had hoped. Almost there. Many weeks, maybe months, had now gone by.

He then wanted the dog to use his nose to force the screen door open. The doctor accomplished this with a command of three eye blinks, and the dog's strong desire to chase after a cat that came around ever so often. The doctor was now ready. He had only to wait for one more thing.

The neighbor soon stopped by again, and as luck would have it, he asked the doctor if he would like some fresh air. The doctor quickly replied with eyeballs moving upwards signifying a "yes." The neighbor opened the heavy sliding glass door to the house and then soon left. NOW the time was right.

The doctor activated the computer voice: "Here, Lucy" and she came running. He then looked heavenward with both eyes and Lucy jumped up higher and higher until she pushed the doctor off of his pedestal. The Head hung there dangling from the eight plastic tubes attached to the mechanical heart. Lucy now saw The Head as a toy and began to paw it, causing it to twist and bounce. The doctor's eyes looked fearful and dizzy. Finally, Lucy began to gnaw at her new toy, pulling on the tubes as they continued to transport the life-sustaining blood. One eventually broke loose and then another, blood spurting everywhere. Good, thought the doctor, it was about time.

Finally, The Head broke free and took a bounce on the floor. Lucy got back down on all fours and found it to be a nice basketball and pushed it around. The doctor was just able to blink twice, causing the pooch to drag him toward the screen door. He then blinked three times and Lucy stuck her nose in the edge of the screen door and pushed it sideways, opening it just enough for her—and hopefully him—to go through.

Lucy eventually made her way through the open screen door with her new toy. The Head rolled onto the deck, but as it approached the edge, Lucy—just at the last moment—stopped the doctor's head from falling over the side. She then gnawed at the nose and one of the ears. Lucy pulled on the detached blood supply tubes as if trying to kill off one of her prey. For the first time, the doctor revealed physical pain in his eyes; one could see the life going out of him. Lucy kicked at it and pushed.

The doctor's head rolled back to the edge of the deck and stopped, his large nose stopping the roll. Lucy walked up and looked down at Dr. Johnson. The doctor's eyes rolled in every direction and Lucy twisted her head in confusion. The doctor looked up at the loyal, loveable dog with penetrating eyeballs and begged her to, "Please, help me."

Lucy lowered her head and pushed on the head with her snout. The head twisted, slowly tipped, rolled over the side, and down it went, bouncing off rock outcroppings until it finally hit the shoreline. With the doctor's eyes still open, waves began washing over his head. There was genuine sadness in this man's eyes.

Bare feet are seen running along the sand, leaving tracks that are quickly washed away by the incoming tide. Young hands then reach down to pick up the doctor's head; his tongue hanging limply from his mouth.

There are the sounds of kids playing in the street and the loud rumble of a boom box from a passing car. A jet flies over with a scream and a boom. A diesel locomotive sounds its horn. A voice calls out "Doctor, doctor, I found your beagle down the street.

"Huh? What?"

Lucy jumped up on the couch, where a man was lying under a blanket on a living room couch, and then aggressively licked his face in joy.

"Lucy! Where have you been?"

The neighbor answered for her: "I guess she got through the fence."

"Damn, you know, Hollis," replied the reclining man, "I was having this crazy dream—that I was a doctor without a body."

"Ha, YOU a doctor!"

Getting Old
Not Guilty By Reason Of
Mental Disease Or Defect
—Hiney Hornblocker, 2016, revised 2022

The Following Article is Fictional and Does Not Represent Any Actual Person or Event—at least none that I can remember.

(JUST MARKING TIME: Some random thoughts that have gone through his mind recently:)

"WARNING: DO NOT READ THIS ARTICLE IF YOU ARE OVER 60 YEARS OF AGE. It is assuredly depressing and can cause sleepless nights and concern for your own wellbeing. Don't read it if you suffer from clinical depression or simply don't want to be dismally despondent at this time."

"If you are miserable, downhearted, dispirited, or downright disconsolate and dejected, then do not read this article. The writer will not be held responsible for any actions taken by the reader that might lead to harm upon himself. If you become discouraged, crestfallen, demoralized, or miserably gloomy, then you should see a doctor as soon as possible. Drugs for every conceivable affliction are now available that promise to solve all your problems, and advertising for them can be seen on television commercials daily—with a phone number to call."

As I, Hiney Hornblocker, approach year 68 of my life on Earth, I begin to "feel" old. It seems I'm now headed on the down side of my life's Ferris Wheel…approaching the ground, approaching mother earth. My swinging seat is hanging over open space and that is quite frightening. The things I had hoped to do someday, well, I now realize are never going to happen. There's not much time left before one reaches the ground…and below it. I reside to that fact with a sigh of desperate sorrow.

Things begin to loose their meaning and my life's purpose up to this point is in question. What good, I ask myself, was my life's work? Who did it really help? What improvements did I make to society? What will I leave behind that people will remember? I know full well that most everything I own or created with my imaginative brain will now be assigned to a grand circular file. What I created, what I collected, what I cared most about, will all be thrown into the city's Dumpster or sold for pennies at a garage sale.

You look at things you've done—accomplishments, home improvements, a successful career—maybe—and think, "It's all over, there is to be no more." Why even wash the car or clean the windows of my house, or even water the lawn? Why leave the house, buy more groceries, go anywhere at all? Sitting in front of the boob tube will just have to do. "No, hell no," I say, "that's not for me," but do I have a choice?

I find it takes longer to get things done; my life seems more jam-packed, "I'm busy as a cat in a barn full of rats," and yet nothing is accomplished as each day whizzes by faster and faster, and... what to Hell, why try to do anything anymore? I used to take a lot of pictures, no reason to do it now. I cancelled all of my magazine subscriptions, no need now to learn anything new. My roof shingles will need replacing soon; no need for them now; a leaky roof only needs a few kitchen pots. I ruminate over the disquieting idea of just sitting and watching television with shoes and socks off and belly hanging out—and how useless to others I will be. The lives of many elderly people become quite lonely when their spouse dies—followed by their pet cat and pet dog—and they begin to mark time, just waiting for the last chore on earth: DEATH...and that's usually not an easy one.

My memory has started to fail me. "Where in the devil did I leave my car keys, the house keys, the keys to my bank box, wait, what bank, for God's sake, is my money in?" In the bank box lays my *Last Will & Testament*, *Power of Attorney*, and *Directive To Physicians* (Hopefully a 'Do Not Resuscitate Order'). I sure wouldn't want a doctor to try to keep me alive in a state of "bedriddenness" as they try to determine whether I had asked legally to be relieved of life's duties. They wouldn't understand, but I'd gladly stop drinking fluids and start taking that soothing morphine…the higher the dose the better.

I can't seem to concentrate anymore. I just stare at the television set not able to remember what had happened in the story before the commercial. Someone tries to tell me a joke and by the time he gets to the punch line, well, I don't laugh because I've forgotten the entire story. I can't even keep track of what day of the week it is.

Then there's a trip to the bathroom with more than regular regularity; they call it "frequent urination." Making numerous trips to the "head" during the night becomes a nightmare of its own. Drinking enough water to avoid dehydration becomes a major effort and I can't ever seem to drink enough, and yet drinking what I should works against a goodnight's rest. Sleep quickly becomes more valuable and a major daily topic of discussion. Dehydration causes weakness, light-headedness, dizziness, even fainting, so I can't win either way.

I find myself obsessing with things, unable to make a decision, waking up in the middle of the night worrying about something I need to do, how to solve a problem, and I don't mean mathematical. I worry about the toilet that keeps cutting on, knowing full well that the flapper needs replacing. I worry about the oil leak from my vehicle and how much it will cost to fix it, especially since the vehicle is over twenty years old and most parts are no longer available. I worry about the young fighting newlyweds living next door and, if, and when, a bullet will penetrate my house. And I worry about the city's daily robberies, shootings at the local convenience stores, and deadly family arguments. Life is becoming like the fruitless reading of a website's contractual agreement: it makes one's head spin! That's why no one reads the agreement, and that's why I just stay home!

I'm disenfranchised. Technology has left me out in the cold: computer, smartphone, Internet, *Twitter*, *Facebook*, driverless cars, wireless everything…but who really needs them? They're for communicating with other human beings, and, as an aging man, that's not what I'm looking for. I want solitude, tranquility… to be left alone.

The new technologies are beginning to muddle my mind. That rhymes. The new must-have gadgets—and I can't program them—at least I don't want to take the inordinate time required to read the detailed instructions just to find the basic "how-to's." And I have no desire to know all the hundreds of other things the device can do. Here's a new digital answering machine and I can't figure out how to record a simple outgoing message! Push this button and that button, pull that switch—it's simply Digital Hell, with the smart televisions, smartphones, smart refrigerators, smart cars, smart homes, and even smart frying pans. (Are they teaching kids in school how to be smart in case these electronic gadgets loose their charge?) I have a digital still camera with a manual that's literally hundreds of pages long—and claims the camera can even shoot video! My patience has left me, it too has had enough. I'm close to throwing something, like this lovely new plastic phone! Hundreds of settings and options; just push this "MENU" button and all of your problems will go away. No, all I want, and need, is a 1950's dial-up telephone! Black or tan.

Watching an old movie or television show is depressing. All the actors you once enjoyed on the big—and small—screen are now old and decrepit. They are, my God, getting frickin' old—I can't be, can I? I was watching a movie channel when they were advertising up-coming movies by showing close-ups of some well-known actors—ones I used to enjoy watching—the trouble was, they were all dead: John Wayne, Marlon Brando, Dean Martin, George C. Scott, Steve McQueen, George Kennedy, Paul Newman, all gone. All of us, even the rich and famous, are here for only a short time.

When watching reruns of old television programs made for the original 1950's 13-inch, 1:1.33, black & white TV screen—programs you watched when you were young—you notice just how simple and primitive they were and just how old the clothes and cars were—*Jack Benny, I Love Lucy, Kojak, Our Gang Comedies, The Beverly Hillbillies, The Dukes of Hazard, Dennis The Menace.* They were not period films when they were made and yet you were there to watch them! Sometimes you can't pay attention to the old reruns because you just focus on those actors that are no longer with us now—just lying there in a rotting wooden coffin with six feet of mother earth above them.

I can't spell words anymore. I'm trying to type an article on my computer. I stare at a word knowing the spelling is incorrect, but can't, for the life-of-me, make it right. A letter transposed or missing all together, something is not right—contrapshun, a common word and I can't spell it! Dissentary, miniskeul, entabliture, zenophobia...what gives?

I can't seem to keep things organized anymore. Simply put, I can't find my stuff and I'm a very organized individual, so what gives? Definitely no living space left. Is this yet another symptom of getting old? "Can't see, can't do," my father used to say when he started wearing bifocals and trying to hammer a nail down straight. It now becomes harder to accomplish something simple. Frustration looms larger. Effort is no longer effortless.

I used to write, but now new thoughts don't come, and when they do, I can't even complete the thought. My brain works at about the speed of *Microsoft Word* when it has been sitting idle for a few minutes on my computer—the speed of an inebriated snail. *Microsoft Word* is no place to record ideas on the fly; I will have forgotten my original thought long before it powers back up (Bill Gates never seemed to care). And I can't remember to carry a small notebook and pencil in my shirt pocket, but even when I do, my valued thought is usually gone by the time I get the notebook out of pocket and pencil in hand. A thought quickly scribbled down was readable, but now I can't even read my own handwriting. Maybe my mind is now just scribbles and kibbles and bits. Yes, getting old is a hard thing to do.

Each day is the same as the last: routine becoming a tiresome bore, the same "old" world-weariness every lousy day. Even today's television programming is boring. It's as repetitive as a mechanical toy teddy bear, and if you don't like cop dramas—those "procedurals"—you're out of luck.

How mundane is it all. I look at life in a whole new light, but it's not uplifting, it's disheartening. Even eating is a chore. No longer anything to look forward to or care about. What I eat, I don't care, just something to survive—a bottle of *Insure* will do just fine. Getting old is trying to finish off your life—closing the deal. There is no conclusion to depression. You're sad, and then you die…alone.

And if one doesn't have a family, he has no purpose, no reason to go on. Again the regimen and routine. The workweek—fifty-two of them every year—each one exactly the same as the last: seven days with a two-day weekend to catch up on house maintenance and family problems. In my case, I never wanted a job that was "routine, and as I get older, I see "routines" happening anyway. Terrible Mondays and Housework Saturdays keep coming up over and over and over again. I'm tired of that routine—the same number of days each year—and I'm even rousted out of bed the same time every morning by barking dogs and chirping birds. *Christmas Eve, Thanksgiving, Halloween, Easter, President's Day*, people's birthdays, all on the same frickin' day every year. We're bred to be like, well, programmed robots to make things we can sell to someone else so we can make just enough money to buy what "they" then want us to buy—a horrendous vicious cycle of wasted time and money.

Yes, I'm tired of solving problems and doing routine maintenance. I have no desire to replace equipment that has plum-quit working like the computer, vacuum cleaner, window air-conditioner, the small-screen television, or even the life-sustaining refrigerator. They can just sit there; I can do without, and instead of calling a plumber, I can just use some duct tape or dig a deep hole in the backyard. If you can dig a deep enough hole, outhouses are not all that bad.

When you're approaching 70, you also find you're just plain tired of doing paperwork, paying taxes, paying bills, and maintaining the unwashed family car (or is it "cars" now that every individual in a family has a vehicle). Your car is leaking oil and antifreeze and maybe *Coca-Cola.* You quit trying to clean up the house, "I'll get to it tomorrow." You're tired of dealing with your grown children who want to move in with you AND bring all their belongings (and their children) with them! Enough already you say, "Get me a one-way ticket to *Siberia* or *Timbuktu.* Some place without cars and kids."

I want to be able to turn on the tap and not worry about how much the gas bill will be or when the water heater will need to be replaced. I don't want to worry about paying still more new taxes of all kinds, getting the roof shingles replaced, or cutting down a dead tree in the front yard before it lands on the house or on my nice car? Does my auto registration need renewing? They'll send me a notice; I'm not to worry. And if they don't, a street cop will surely let me know. I wouldn't much care for a stretch in the hoosegow, though I would appreciate the free room and board!

All motivation is lost, no energy, no inspiration. I don't want to be anywhere. I feel distant even in my own bedroom—no importance to my environment, my collected things—meaninglessness to it all. Everywhere is nowhere. I'm just tired of the world around me and it all feels foreign and useless, and I'm ready to let someone else deal with it.

You lose interest in keeping up with family and friends; you just want peace and quiet, not more tasks and problems to deal with. You loose interest in all of your unfinished projects and things you had hoped to accomplish. Even travel—the vacation trips you had hoped to make—now become just something you must strive to forget about.

You put on a piece of clothing and suddenly remember that a friend or relative had given it to you, and then you realize, and are crestfallen to know, that he or she is no longer with the living.

I'm tired of going to retail outlets. Racks and racks and racks of stuff in pretty packages—most of which we have no need of; just the incessant advertising has made us think we do. How different are those many brands of soap, just the aroma I suspect?

How many kinds of toilet paper? Not about the aroma I'm sure. And then there's the mall and store music blasting continuously to sooth and mesmerize; lulling us into making a purchase—and making it inevitable for you to end the year in debt.

Before age 70, one's life seems quite long. My summers as a kid seemed to last forever and I was even looking forward to the new school year, but now, a year of one's life passes much too quickly; every week, every year, getting noticeably shorter. If you are retired with nothing to do, maybe that's a good thing, but with each day passing in a twinkling of the eye, the work accomplished is less, much less. Your physical body is also moving slower, much slower, like a robot running low on battery power. Even getting out of bed is sluggish with staggering multiple trips to the bathroom during the night a routine endeavor. When getting old you expect your body to slow down, but your brain gelling, you don't expect that.

As one approaches the ripe young age of 70, there's a new heightened awareness of one's environment. You notice people's chiseled and creviced faces. You notice their body's structure: thin, overweight, or obese. You notice the neighborhood with its rows and rows of almost identical houses. You notice tree roots that have buckled a section of sidewalk and are waiting—almost a dare—for you to trip and break something. You notice a homeless man with a military backpack and a scruffy dog trailing behind him and you think, 'that could be me so very soon.'

You notice the acres and acres of retail businesses from horizon to horizon that have replaced our corn and wheat fields—as many of our foodstuffs are now imported from other countries. You look at the roadways, bridges and strip centers in the country and think how monotonous it all is. I walk the streets with my dog and observe only shopping centers with acres of concrete, flashing neon signs, fast food trash bags, beer cans strewn merrily about, and automobiles zipping by incessantly.

Cookie-cutter houses—even the ones costing a half-million or more—cover the landscape with barely any air space between them. From the air, one sees only miles and miles in every direction of asphalt shingles. It looks more like some lunar landscape of desolation. I look at a relatively new parking lot or highway now covered with cracked asphalt because the thickness of the asphalt had been cut in half by the city government from the engineer's requirements and little or no rebar and wire mesh was put in the concrete work. This is the world we've built.

Television. Everything seems so artificial. Like watching a film on the new 3D televisions—wow, awesome, but not real. Cars zipping by, houses just sitting there inert like a movie set. The few kids seen outside walk with their heads down, earphones stuck in their hearing organs and looking at their mobile phone. It's an almost indescribable feeling, but I will try anyway. The constant repetition of events—like political ads, weather reports, advertising in general—is like being mesmerized by a flashing streetlight or clicking turn arrow. The big, flat television of today adds to the effect as it sits there dominating the room with its dynamic, fast-paced images. And it's not just the television, it's the whole room—the furniture, decoration, framed art, collectibles—all become just a big sheet of wallpaper. My stuff has been there for many years, mostly untouched, not even dusted; a three-dimensional reality lost on me. It's like an art museum of hanging art that you just quickly walk past.

You pay more attention to the weather, the city traffic, the cannonade of commercials that seem like a three-dimensional video game that's closing in on you—inundating, assailing. You are strapped to a chair and forced to watch thousands of almost continuous, fast-paced commercials. It's enough to make you want to scream—or smash the television screen with your remote control. Are commercials the happy result of 300 years of progress in America? You look at the worth of things. The media promotes what is not important: big flat-screen TV's, food processors, "healthy" foods, the biggest of SUV's, and the million or so fast-food restaurants. You find yourself loosing interest in the "things" you once enjoyed working on...nothing, at least over the air, is entertaining anymore. "Honey, I'm turning the frickin' television off...and unplugging it!"

Yes, instead of looking out the window to see the world, we see it on a large flat-screen television. The only connection to the outside world is a computer, smartphone, or lowly television antennae. There's also the staring—and sometimes yelling—at someone through a car window when they cut you off. The invention of central air-conditioning must have started it all; no longer do residents sit on the front porch and say "hi" to their neighbors—a few do. And their houses are wrapped in chain link fences or six-foot-tall cedar fences, or both.

I look at the television screen and see presentations that are carefully scripted and professionally photographed and they all appear quite artificial, just millions of changing pixels on flickering boob tubes. I can't just enjoy the show, I see beyond it. In a television drama, I ignore the story and look at the set lighting and the actor's performances—not the characters in the episode. I don't get lost in the story. Where's the suspense sufficient enough to get involved in the plot? The story doesn't even build in intensity. Don't get me wrong, some episodes do grip me, but they are a rarity these days. With the news, I turn off the sound and watch a news anchor as he reads the teleprompter. It seems as if I'm watching a sci-fi space movie; he looks like an alien robot. Maybe he's just a one-dimensional digital image. With all that makeup, how do you know he's not? (Young Japanese inventors are working hard to replace Homo Sapiens.) You can talk to your cell phone and it will respond. And then there's the murder and mayhem on dramatic television that has become all too real with this country's actual crime and murder at an all-time high. Is there any connection between the two, the watching of television and the killing of people?

Television programs—especially the free "over-the-air" offerings fed by a *Radio Shack* antennae on the roof—are chock full of nothing but old people, especially on the so-called "news" programs—*ABC, NBC, CBS,* and even *PBS*—where the so called "journalists" have been there for forty years or more, but still able to read the teleprompter that displays an associate's prepared text. I wonder how big the font is? There must be only three or four words per line!

Do you feel you're watching television programs intended for old people, every network trying to sell you on a heavy-duty drug that will cure what ails the "senior citizen." *Alzheimer's*, high blood pressure, kidney disease, diabetes, potbelly syndrome, crooked toe, erectile dysfunction…oh, my God, medicines that will solve all our health problems, and then some claim they enhance family fun, friendships, and fertility—how wonderful!

One third of every hour addresses the ailments of old people—life-threatening ailments: like a leg too short, frightening bad odor, or dangerously long hangnails. I really must already be dead after hearing what horrors ail me! "If you have a sudden drop in blood pressure, call your doctor right away. Bad back, sore feet? We've got the answer for you. Do you have arthritis, mesothelioma, psoriasis, or callused feet? Well, of course you do, you must, you're almost a silver-headed 70! "We have just the thing for you: a wheelchair and someone to push you around. The government will finance it, don't you worry! We know you must have wrinkled skin, enlarged blue veins, a balding head, and a very crooked big toe. Call us now!" We must listen to this hard sell eighteen minutes out of every confounded hour! We must listen to all the health warnings by the off-camera narrator if we decide to tackle this wondrous drug. The voice warns of far worse health problems than the mild disorder you may have started with. "Why is this marvelous medical breakthrough, Big Pharma's *ZisWillMakeYouLoose,* just for me?" you ask. Anyone else got that problem? Loose bowels. One only needs to stop the hamburger and T-bone steak and try some oatmeal, hot chocolate, cream corn, a vegetable salad, and maybe a prune or two.

You look at how this country has changed and it doesn't look pretty. For example, a very-large national company pushes cows onto a long stainless steel conveyor belt and out comes a pallet of boxed, precooked, frozen hamburger patties ready to be shipped thousands of miles to grocery chains and fast-food restaurants around the country. *McDonalds*, with its "Speedee Service System,"—begun in 1940—was it the beginning of our obese, salt-infested society? No wonder America is so overweight. Just read the saturated fat and cholesterol percentages on any grocery store product. Fruits and fresh vegetables are now the only option.

And then there's the instructions on plastic food packaging that inevitably fails to work: *"Easy Open—Just Pull Apart And Enjoy," "Easy Open Notch,"* or *"Tear Here >"* with the arrow pointing to a structurally reinforced plastic seal. Good luck tearing it there. Even a new roll of fluffy white toilet paper is hard to unravel. The outer layers are adhered somehow so when you try to pull or carefully start the roll, it tears into numerous layers thus ripping the roll to shreds. Who designs this stuff anyway? A third-grade kid in Pakistan who doesn't even know what toilet paper is?

Impatience: I'm loosing patience with things. It's no longer effortless to place a letter into an envelope, a book into an overcrowded bookshelf, or a bulbous pillow back into its case. Things fall off shelves that I seem to be just standing near, I haven't even touched! The refrigerator is crowded, so I'm not surprised things fall out, and my desk is inundated with papers, pencils & pens, books, folders, rubber stamps, a weight scale, a pencil sharpener, and several old telephones. No wonder things mysteriously jump to the floor.

My impatience and irritability with things—and people—is growing with age. I twiddle my thumbs and tap my feet as I try desperately to remain calm. My blood pressure rises, 130, 140, 150. I grow exhausted waiting for something to happen. The weeds grow six-foot tall in an alley that's pot-marked with all manner of refuse. Dogs and foraging cats by the hundreds run loose in the neighborhood. Dog's yelp incessantly at night and cats leave the feathers of conquered birds in the backyard. Everything beeps: the cell phone, microwave, the computer's email. Where's the peace and quiet in retirement? Can it only be found in a nursing home? No, trust me, it doesn't happen there! You've got nurse assistants waking you up to dispense meds throughout the day—and night—and others trying to get you to eat or go for a wheelchair ride to soak up some sunlight.

I also get impatient with people who do stupid things—like tying very short, six-foot or less, thirty-pound chains in their backyard so they can't move about; the dogs that is. And where dogs never see a human until a bowl of dry dog food is brought to them in the evening. I lose patience with people putting at risk the young children walking or riding down the sidewalk by blocking their way with a parked vehicle. This obstacle forcing the kids to turn out into the street in order to circumnavigate the vehicle, causing them to ride in front of an oncoming car. Wake up people! My degree of impatience with something or someone irritating me has gradually increased so that a dangerous confrontation with someone is now more likely. People throwing trash out their car windows or people illegally putting out bandit signs like *"We Buy Crappy Houses,"* or *"No Dinero Down,"* or *"Astronaut Wanted For Free Trip To Moon."* I think I'll start carrying handcuffs to arrest these code compliance violators. A driver cutting me off as he tries to exit from an outside lane is enough to make me want to take action against the offending party. I want to intentionally side swipe his car to leave a nicely scraped-up paint job. Maybe that'll get him to slow down. Even the computer I have used for many things over many years is beginning to irritate me. It's harder to track down a document, install application updates, learn a new app without a 200-page digital instruction manual, and it even takes longer to shut off the computer. I'm thinking I'll turn it off for the last time and enjoy a little peace. The computer will fit just fine in the city's Dumpster.

Everything is automated today. Communication through email, voicemail, online webites—all simply inhuman. When you try to connect with someone online or by telephone to resolve a problem or make a doctor's appointment, you get small-print text or some monotonous-voiced robot. So I would just like to quit going to doctors, the dentist, the bank, the pharmacy…just about everywhere.

Speaking of the computer, I'm just bombarded by junk emails (a beep every few seconds) and on the telephone recorded voices with no one to yell back at, how unfair. Getting put on the national

"Do Not Call" list doesn't stop the intrusions. Responding directly to them with "Please stop sending me your frickin' ads" only encourages them to call back. And writing to your congressman doesn't help, of course, so I think it's time to bomb some Chinese and Pakistani companies. When you try to unsubscribe from an e-mail ad, you get "We're sorry to see you go." Oh, I'm sure, a potential loss of business. What sorrow I feel! I'm heartbroken. I think I'll just sign back up. I love getting all those unwanted e-mails, the more the merrier, the more wasted time in my now quickly diminishing life span. Even an abruptly ringing telephone is an annoyance; my level of stress instantly elevated—and if you dare to answer it, there's more bad news, gargantuan problems to deal with. Things breaking down and needing to be fixed upset me; just more "crap" to deal with. Enough, already! And there are the living telemarketers (not robots) calling at dinnertime. If I can just get rid of them there will be some peace and quite so I can get something productive and useful accomplished. Shut everything down I'm thinking, "no computer, no phone, and no damn electricity to complicate my life."

And speaking of electricity, what would happen if *Ohm's Law* (I=V/R) were suddenly to change on this planet? Chaos, that's what! Nothing electronic would work. No vehicles in motion, no lights indoor or out, no television or radio broadcasts, no internet, no cell phones, no water pumping stations or gas pumps. No trucks hauling groceries, no mail service, and all factories shut down…mayhem! A total collapse of this world's developed civilizations. The third world countries might now be back on an equal footing. We'd all have to go into survival mode and invent things all anew—a whole new set of routines! Plant our own seeds to grow, and harvest our own food. Horses and wagons for transportation. Boredom to the wind!

What's the worth of it all? I have a desire to shut down all connections to the outside—the world that resides beyond my house's interior—with the phone and the internet shut down, the front door locked, lights off. A weird feeling is coming over me, no desire to go on—why should I do anything? I made a white business card that's printed in it's four corners with: *No Phone*,

No Address, *No Email*, and *No Facebook*, and in the center is written *"No Name."* That's me.

I'm mad, I'm angry, and I'm fed up. The federal government is frickin' out of control! Neither the far-left democrats nor the bought-and-paid-for republicans can be trusted. It's clear they don't work for the people. No term limits on congressmen. They're secure in their jobs for decades and get a full pension for life after just six years in office! You've heard that all before, but what's different? It's my patience that's out of control. New Zealand is looking better all the time. Nineteen trillion dollars in debt to be paid back by the American people even when the interest rates on our personal savings are less than one percent! Where's the hope? What's the use? Where's the opposite of neurological stress? Even the ballot box can no longer be trusted. There's a sadness and hopelessness in my heart that mankind, and our government, have not advanced one iota toward a better world of peace and cooperation. Maybe a long, deep toke on a water pipe will solve the problem.

I've watched the value of money go down the proverbial toilet, if not literally. I remember when a twenty-dollar bill provided all the necessities for a month. College tuition was $400 a semester—and that included room and board. Job salaries and social security payments certainly haven't kept up with inflation. And property taxes, income taxes, and sales taxes…it's a wonderment that the government hasn't taken our first born for a lifetime of conscription. We may not realize it, but slavery is back…for ALL the races now.

Loss. Many persons around you, old friends from a near and distant past, are suddenly acquiring a serious illness that will shorten their life span: cancer, *Alzheimer's, Parkinson's*, vascular dementia, cardiovascular diseases, or a violent, unexpected, traffic accident. Many die sooner than later. And some of these "before-their-time" deaths, you realize, have actually been caused by their own doctor—late in getting a prescription drug to a patient for an infection, overdosing a patient, giving the patient anything they want, or often, simply miss-diagnosing the problem.

You think about the friends and family who died before their time, long before. They had lots of plans for their approaching retirements and then—suddenly—a killer disease and it was all over. One of my first cousins "acquires" a minor chest pain that turns out to be a cancer that quickly went to one kidney and then to the other and then led to a mild stroke that left him speechless and unable to write or practice his trade. Another first cousin is violently beat to near death with a fireplace poker by his teen-age daughter and her boyfriend—and then they bury him while he's still alive! Unfortunately, he choked on dry dirt and didn't recover from his shortness of breath. And my mother was given a heavily advertized product (*Boniva*) by her doctor for an illness she didn't even have, only to cause her a stroke while she was dancing, and that quickly killed her stone dead. (Sally Field— *The Flying Nun*—ceased mysteriously touting this osteoporosis drug just three weeks after my mother had taken just one *Boniva* tablet.)

As we approach the upper region of our life spans, the death of family members and friends becomes quite traumatic. As one ages, rare photos of himself taken by others, and images of family members and friends in the distant past, become more precious. They're heartwarming or invoke the sadness of happy times lost. You miss all the pets you had in the past. It even hurts to the lowest ventricle of your heart to see a plant or tree or animal that is dying. All living things still walking about, or blowing in the wind, seem to be of even more importance.

There's death all around you, your family, friends, and pets. It's hard to see animals injured or killed. I now seem to be more emo-tionally affected, "a terrible loss," I think. I don't even have to know them to experience grief.

I walk through *Pick-n-Pull*, an auto graveyard with literally thousands of vehicles that have been scavenged of engine parts, wheels, door handles, transmissions—and I feel a terrible sense of loss...the end of life of an inanimate object is almost as sad as that of a human's. Or is it that a human's death is simply no more important than those inanimate objects? Either way, when you're no longer useful, you're destined for the salvage yard.

All the people you've known that have passed through your life, in a way, you miss them all. You stay in, reclusive, because you don't want to meet new people; you don't want to add any new horses to the stables. You see these friends as distant, disconnected, their faces fading into the yonder.

When your dog becomes your best—and sometimes only— devoted and trusted friend, you find yourself crawling back into the warm womb of your home, with no desire to keep in touch with anyone. "Just leave me alone," you would like to say to them, and to help stem the intrusions, you want to pull the cord from the phone jack on the wall.

You think about the things in your life that, if you had done differently, might have changed your direction in life. Just five or six different decisions, that's all, then what would have been the outcome? Oh, for a second chance. A job you took—or didn't. Or giving up on an idea too soon. A piece of Real Estate you could have bought quite inexpensively, but didn't, and it became worth millions of dollars just a few years later! Or maybe a decision you made not to advance your formal education any further. Maybe your choice of spouse. How might your life have been different... or maybe not.

Unrealized dreams. There are so many things you wanted to do, but are drastically waning in desire and opportunities. You see an auto junkyard with acres and acres of rusting, bent up bodies with parts ripped-out. You see acres and acres of cemeteries. You think, "how is this world better for us having been here?" Many species have gone extinct on this here planet; maybe it's our turn to go. Better for the planet, to be sure.

Veterinarians give pets a far more thorough physical examination than do the doctors of humans. Doctors used to check the eyes, ears, hands, the heart rhythm, and even tapped on the knees checking for normal reflexes, but they check nothing now, absolutely nothing; they just ask you why you came to see them. "I feel fine," I reply, "but I can't tell what ails me just by looking in my bathroom mirror." "Need any meds?" the doctor asks, and I respond, "Well, what have you got? Anything medicinal? A kilo of marijuana, maybe?"

You look at a national, highly touted, football game and realize just how primitive an activity it is. Men with steal helmets, heavy shoulder pads and knee pads, all just fighting over a leather ball— one tribal band trying to wrestle the ball away from the other— and it's not even a foodstuff. They're just tussling with each other in front of millions to get a very big monthly paycheck. They're also guaranteed to have permanently damaged brain matter. Our military soldiers, who also wear metal "piss pots," and fight for "freedom," make only peanuts. Or how about that bunch of min-imally dressed, long-legged men, kicking a ball around a large green plastic-grassed field, often using their hard head to move the ball? "Soccer," I think they call it. Why not "Sockhim?"

Planes, trains, and automobiles. Nature is alive and well— somewhere—but it's besieged by the harsh sounds of our urban environment: jets flying over, blaring boom-boxes, diesel locos blasting their thundering horns incessantly with hundreds of freight cars rumbling tediously behind, and the cursed clanging at railroad crossings—all so brutally irritating, and building in me an internal psychological stress. On freeways, automobiles scramble at 70-plus miles per hour as if in a race to a *Grand Prix* finish line. A fire station near my house supplies the daily howling of ladder trucks and the piercing cry out of blue-lighted ambulances. And then there are the pounding semi-trucks and screaming motorcycles of city life with earthmovers at construc-tion sites groaning and growling. And the dump trucks, *FedEx* vans, *UPS*, *Amazon Prime*, and speeding autos barreling down residential streets creating the painfully high decibels that are sure to destroy eardrums. No wonder everyone keeps his home's windows shut tight with an air conditioner rumbling and spitting even on cool, crisp days.

Just trying to file papers like bank statements is a depressing chore. Relieving oneself is an adventure. You become more aware of your environment and are irritated by your own basic bodily functions and the increased time it takes to deal with them. Stated simply: as you grow older, your bodily functions dictate your daily life.

One becomes disassociated with the world around him. The people, places and things all seem so inconsequential. Not part of your world anymore. You're now above it all, of no concern to you. All of it seems otherworldly: the physical environment, the animals, the insects, and your fellow Homo Sapiens. I can't imagine a *FedEx* deliveryman or *U.S.* Postman saddled with the same task over and over and over again throughout his working life. An alarm clock waking one from a sound sleep the same time every day, every week, every blasted year for maybe half a lifetime. What's the use? The only way they can survive is having interesting, engaging hobbies…or kids they're always having to break out of jail.

I watch the many living things on this here planet trying to make a go of it, from colorful butterflies dancing around trumpet vines, to boisterous squirrels and sneaky little rats, and I don't understand why we humans should think we're so special. We developed over millions of years just as all of the other creatures on this planet did, and so the sexual dances and reproductive systems are all quite similar.

As we get older, life is reduced to sitting for untold hours watching 1950's and '60's television shows like *Roy Rogers, Bonanza, The Beverly Hillbillies, Johnny Carson, Leave It To Beaver, The Munsters*; at least that's what some of my friends are doing. But not me, no way, Jose! How about Perry *Mason, Petticoat Junction,* and *The Adams Family*—all great shows, but give me an effin' break!

There's something in the air, like the eerie feeling one gets in a heavy fog bank. The sun is up there, you know that for sure, but the life-sustaining rays aren't quite reaching you. Is this the new normal? Is this just getting flamin' old? Is this an intentional way to sap the remaining life out of you?

I now live in a world where the sun rarely comes out. Enthusiasm for anything is gone. Depression is like a dark, drizzly, sunless day that never seems to end, and that's what seems to be happening to me: despondency, lack of energy, a bottom-of-the-well sadness. There appears to be no future, so I'm becoming reclusive…and worse, I come to like it. I'll have to unplug my phone so it won't ring and interrupt my sorely needed peace.

Why even get up in the morning? The effort is immensely tiresome and requires strenuous physical and mental exertion. I become exhausted just cogitating about what I have to do that day even when it's just more of the confounded same. Why bother to get out of that comfortable bed? Why get dressed, put on socks, wash my teeth—why for heaven sakes, why? Confounded why?

My life is a clicking, ticking clock. Tick tock, tick tock, sixty times a dad-gum minute like an antique self-winding timepiece, over and over and over again. Tick, tick, tick, time passing and yet standing so eerily still.

You notice a tree, that was once just a young sapling, now growing through a rusty chain-link fence and think, "that tree's going to win the battle with that old wire fence, just like old age is going to win the battle over my fearfully diminishing life span."

As one gets older, he acquires a wider view of the world through the lives of other people. You meet and get to know more and more fellow humans in many walks of life and thus you gain new useful knowledge through assimilation. But now, how do you put it to use in your waning years? Everyone in the professional world seems younger than yourself—your doctor, your lawyer, your chiropractor, and your favorite loony-tunes psychic—many with multiple professional degrees and yet they look like nothing more than college kids. Professionals used to be older, more experienced, more mature, to be looked up to, but now just out of grade school?—how weird! (Well, except for career politicians— they're as old as the earth itself.) The movie stars I once worked alongside in the film business, upon seeing them now in a recent movie, all look so damned old! And the friends I haven't seen in scores of years—all look so elderly in appearance! Wrinkled, blotched skin, sagging faces, and drooping eyes. No, it can't be happening to me, can it?

When my doctor handed me a plastic multi-lidded pillbox with some colored beads to see if I could take my own medications, well, that's when I knew it was all over but the crying. Did I really look or act that alone in years?

The hands on a clock move faster and faster as we get older and older, and less seems to get done. You feel your time is running out like the digital timer on a microwave oven; you watch it—stare at it—as it counts down to zero.

What do I do with all of my "stuff?" All of no real value to me now, and probably to no one else. My life's work, what indeed, is it all worth? If I'm not already a famous person and no family to pass it onto, then what are my personal accomplishments all about? My art, photography, written works, hand-made houses, here today gone tomorrow. What do I do with my stamp and coin collection? All of my framed pictures and artwork? All of my antique furniture pieces, grandma's china? If one has plenty of descendants, that's not a worry (unless you abhor them all), but if you have no one to pass it on to, what then? Maybe somewhere there's a heritage museum that will take it all in? I can only hope. A garage sale or estate sale is not an option. I don't get a return on my investment if I figure my original cost, inflation, street value, and many years of storage costs! Only the estate sale vender makes a killing. I might have some collections that would be appreciated by a roadside museum, not lost to oblivion if they had been sold out of a garage. *The Roy Rogers Museum* collection was sadly sold piecemeal after Roy died. All of us aging Rogers fans were dying off and the younger generations didn't give a care, not a hoot. I reckon that's life...and death.

Getting old engenders sagging bodies with overreaching bellies, staggering or limping movements, and aching foot problems of so many varieties that doctors specialize in them. You get up slower, walk slower, and the visiting children and grandkids are just a chore, no longer a welcome interlude. Thankfully, I don't have any.

As you get older, your skin becomes fragile by just looking at it, it peels away and bleeds. You think, "how could this be, I barely touched it?" Every cut of the epidermis now gets infected no matter how small, and you can't lick the wound like a dog would do, to apply an antiseptic. Your wounds never really heal: scabs stay around forever and a permanent skin discoloration remains. One needs to keep the triple antibiotic handy. Maybe you're getting a skin cancer. Look up "Hair Follicle Infections."

As you approach 70, uncontrolled flatulence becomes such a big issue, and is quite embarrassing—or maybe not (at my age what do I care, let them sniff and snicker). And there are now many more trips running to the "head." Your walking has slowed; tripping on an uplifted sidewalk expansion joint is becoming a real possibility. Getting old is so wonderful.

Your days are filled with things to do, but not what you'd like to do. Your chain-link fence is falling down, the living-room carpet faded and unraveling, your antique *Maytag* washing machine rusting flakes of iron oxide and habitually leaking water or some other such fluid: oil maybe, grease, urine? There's no end to the failure of equipment, well, maybe one shouldn't expect them to last fifty years like you had hoped; you have to be happy with two or three. Now days, auto batteries are good only three to five years. My house and yard are beginning to look like the rest of the neighborhood, like "*Sanford & Son Salvage.*" But what do I care now. Someone else can clean it up after I'm dead and buried…or me and my house burned into a pile of brown ashes.

Multi-lane roads and interchanges are expanding throughout the city; a massive spaghetti of roads with multi-layered interstate intersections and millions and millions of vehicles moving from one place to another each and every day—well, a few less on Christmas mornings. How assembly-line like is our world? We're all just cogs in a massive machine…and it makes what, exactly? In a movie theatre's public restroom, there's a long row of white urinals hanging on a ceramic-tiled wall, and all are in use by the patrons who have just left a dark theatre. They're all unzipping, reaching, grabbing. We've all become herds of boisterous chimpanzees as if scrambling to a feeding. Millions of people bustling about from here to there and back again, over and over and over again. Let's face it; we're just a humongous herd of aardvarks. Eating ants and termites? Well, maybe chocolate candy and beefy burgers.

Yes, getting old. No need anymore for cell phones, smart phones, computers, email. Let us old folks proudly carry a business card that says: "I don't do drugs and I don't drink. At my age, I can get the same effect by standing up too fast." Or it might read: "I've finally reached the wonder years. I wonder where I parked my car. I wonder where I left my cell phone. I wonder where my glasses are. And I always wonder what day it is." Better yet, a business card that says simply "*Soon Gone and Forgotten.*"

Roller coaster weather, bumper-to-bumper traffic, plumbing breakdowns, and irritatingly bothersome neighbors are like dynamic, expanding wallpaper patterns slowly closing in on me. I feel inundated—strafed by WWII fighter-bombers that seize me of my sanity.

An elderly lady in a nice suburban neighborhood was fed up with her neighbor who was always feeding the wild deer. That sustenance drew hoards of them that trampled her front lawn, and fertilized it. Maybe they were providing some nutrition to encourage a healthy green lawn, but she found that she had to walk carefully when mowing her own yard. Well, having had enough, the ticked-off lady decided to pick up the gooey refuse and throw it over her neighbor's backyard fence hoping they would get the message, hoping their kids would play in it and track it into THEIR house. Don't know how that came out. And then there was the guy who was fed up with the illegal, neighborhood-polluting "bandit signs" that are stapled to telephone poles and planted on public right-of-ways. The New Home developers and the "*We Buy Ugly Houses*" are the biggest, most successful lawbreakers. Finally, the man had had enough and drove around on Saturday mornings pulling them up and then calling the city to pick up his latest collection. Then there was the 72-year-old gentleman who was tired of drivers cutting him off when they changed lanes, or turned in front of him after an intersection's signal light had already turned red. Fed up, he finally quit trying to break or steer clear of them, just kept his speed, and let them hit him. His car was bent up, but the other guys got traffic tickets. The point is, when you get to a certain age, you won't put up with crap anymore...even at your own peril.

Today's Society.

Commercials. Is this the result of 300 years of progress in America? No? So what is? It may be the powerful, money-hungry companies that produce high-definition full-color commercials designed to convince us to give up every last penny of our meager wealth. Over-the-air television is now nothing but bothersome, unyielding commercials. Maybe no one else feels this, but I think, "Enough already! Why should I go on? For what end?" If you go to a movie theatre now days they show you fifteen minutes of commercials before the show begins; you're paying to see commercials!

Yes, America's commercials, I'm tired of them. All the time, everywhere. They eat one third of airtime and destroy the continuity of a television program that otherwise might have been watchable. No wonder cable networks like *Netflix*—that have no commercials—are gaining dramatically in popularity. We interact with television instead of the real world, instead of our neighbors. And the commercials, they all seem so laughable. We are just numbers—millions of us—easy marks in a mass marketing scheme. Television shows are designed to take our money, providing just enough "entertainment" to hold our attention while they extract every last dollar from our wallet. Dramatic television programs are obviously carefully scripted; commercials are carefully scripted; and sadly, the news is also carefully scripted.

And how much can a person take of the irritating commercial television promises: "It's free for everyone," "No money down," "Quick and easy," "Let the real you shine through," (Oh, great, the real me!) "Injury lawyers available 24/7, nights and weekends!" Wow, I stubbed my toe in the dark of night, who can I sue? "We promise you our best prices!" "Today we're offering an incredible deal!" "Tell your doctor if you have a history of suicidal thoughts." (Damn, I guess I'm going to have to get an appointment, see what they can do for me—probably a concrete cell with steel bunk bed and three squares.)

Programming. I abhor the barrage of commercials that are successfully influencing the buying decisions of millions. You walk into a mammoth warehouse like *Wal-Mart* with acres of strategically displayed housewares, most of which you don't really need, and wonder why? You feel ill. You realize people—especially of a younger age—aren't thinking for themselves anymore. And the media bias makes me realize that honesty, integrity, truth and reality, are all "out the window" in this society. *Twitter, FaceBook, YouTube*, and *Instagram* are the new media—the new source for "factual" information. There's an "underworld" of *Karl Marx* ideals (a classless society run by a dictator) followed by the young generation as the result of intense, progressive high school and college educations. It's no longer just about teaching a trade, but a long-term goal to convert the country to socialism. Big government, societal woes. Why is an aging person concerned about what is happening to this country? He's going to be gone, kaput, of no consequences very soon. Maybe "it's his generation's fault that the country has gone down the toilet," but more likely, he sees that his own life has simply been a waste; his life's work all for naught—to be sold off at a garage sale.

Even the national news has become such a fabrication. There's a complete loss of trust in the information they put out. They don't report the facts; they just export hours and hours of commentary in an effort to tell us what we should think. They apparently don't hire journalists and investigative reporters anymore; just pretty, heavily made up human-like mannequins programmed to read a teleprompter. I watch this and see fact and fiction merging together. There's no reality anymore, no truths. Everything aired is there to influence you, to get you to behave in a certain way. Programming on the old 1950's black & white television set looked and felt distinctly separate from the real world, but that's not the case today and the "news" does a great job of blurring fact with fiction.

When will the major television networks loose all of their dwindling market share is anyone's guess. Parents used to complain about the quality of programming, but made no effort to prevent their children from affixing themselves to the flickering, image-making contraption. But the big-screen television is going away, and all peoples of all ages are now glued securely to the new smartphones for many hours each and every day. What future lives will these people have?

You look at news commentators on the so-called "news" shows like *PBS News Hour, Meet The Press,* and *This Week*—and you see them as robotic figures assigned to that network to disrupt the peace; creating conflict and division with comments about how everything is wrong with, well, everything.

And then there is the repetition of meaningless phrases repeated over and over in the public media. The national news wins the awards for this and the local news comes in second: "We'll give you the latest information as it becomes available." *"More Real News,"* is CBS's actual motto! Why not *"ALL Real News."* And "We'll be right back," is heard before every confounded commercial. And, as it turns out, "right back" really means a seemingly endless 4-1/2 minutes of advertising, and "We're only minutes away from the game" actually means that it's at least 75 minutes before the next football game starts. Yes, I clocked it! Where's the reality—and integrity—these days? The media is not even honest with the mottos they use at the opening of their shows. They should instead say, for example: ABC: *"No News is Good News"* and NBC: *"We Sell Fiction,"* but the winning mottos go to CBS: *"World News Never," "The Myth Makers," "We're The Experts At Speculation,"* or *"CBS Original Reporting: The Latest From Twitter."*

Speaking of reality: television's scripted "reality" shows for the millennials, like the *"Ninja Warrior," "The Voice," "America's Got Talent,"* or *"Big Brother,"* are such wonderful educational entertainment! Just awesome! Don't you just love *"And You Think You Can Dance?"* and *"The Bachelor"*? I'm waiting on pens and needles for the new series, *"Fun In The Sandbox," "How Many Hours Can You Spend On Your Smartphone?"* and *"So You Want To Be President"* hosted by Donald Trump.

And the media is changing our relationships with each other. We get to see open sex, indiscriminant gun use, violent deaths and bloody dead bodies laid out in a bed or on the floor—so common in shows like *Law & Order, Special Victims, Criminal Minds, Chicago P.D., CSI,* and on and on and on. And to think this is not affecting the youth of this country. After watching a couple of violent shows on evening television and then turning on the news, it seems now, the news is even more dramatic and horrifying than the fictional television. And sadly, we're dumbed-down by it all.

There's an intense, magnified nature about me—a heightened awareness of earth's beauty—white cumulous clouds billowing below deep-blue skies, a magnificent red-sky sunset, a cool refreshing breeze, a warm invigorating sun, and joyfully-tweeting birds (and I don't mean prisoners with smartphones). I even find my sense of smell magnified immeasurably. I'm more attuned to the odorous environment, but I don't understand why. Why does my environment seem amplified?

But also stamped in my mind, is the stark ugliness of one's built environment and some of the people who inhabit it: the inconsiderate murderers, belligerent drunk drivers, bandit sign planters, and dangerous buffoons exceeding the neighborhood speed limit by a factor of two. You're consciously trying to slow down and throttle back, fully aware that you're not as alert or energized by daily life as you once were. Your reactions are slower. In fact, who knows, maybe you'll step on the gas when searching for the brake petal! Some of my neighbors have done just that...with the result they rear-ended a car ahead of them or crashed through a chain-link fence and into another's living room. I hope not to do that, but I guess age 70 is the turning point requiring you to be more keenly aware of your environment.

The sun is setting and I'm cruising down a multi-lane freeway and I see before me literally thousands of white-hot headlights rushing toward me in the oncoming lanes. There's a ring of humid air circling each headlight, fog is building, but suddenly, just ahead of me, rows and rows of red taillights get brighter and the vehicles screech to a stop in a chain reaction of burning rubber and out-of-control heart palpitations. Humanity is now subservient to all manner of machine. Your life is in a machine's hands. This country is built by, formed by, controlled by…contraptions.

A cool crisp night outdoors is somehow invigorating. Looking at a clear night sky with bright stars makes one realize he is standing on a tiny planet in a very big mysterious universe. Very sobering. It makes one realize just how small he is—not necessarily insignificant—but he is just one creature among millions. If you lay outside for a time, you can see the stars moving together in a magnificent curve. Do you feel uplifted and joyous or simply dejected? Why does an aging person look up at the stars? With age comes a renewed awareness; a new appreciation for what he's had and has, but also an awareness that one is getting old and time is quickly running out.

A reflection on my life. I fondly remember buying candy in a five & dime store with its well-worn wood-strip flooring and oval island display racks with unpackaged products organized in glass dividers. I remember sitting outside on tables just in front of an outdoor movie screen watching an Elvis Presley movie and later, watching a 70mm wide-screen film: *2001: A Space Odyssey*. The point? The farming town of Kirby, Texas was once a town that stood on its own, but then a nearby city that called itself San Antonio grew and grew and grew until it swallowed up Kirby—incorporating it as a large city usually does—but actually bypassing it, leaving it rundown with a few chickens and goats left behind. It's now a mixed-use neighborhood, both residential and tired commercial businesses sitting side by side. There's *Billy Bob's* auto junkyard and *Brenda's Used Tires* sitting next to *Cling Ling's Chinese Grocery* and next to that a tiny church of unknown denomination. It all seems quite strange that when right next to it, literally feet away, is a multi-lane interstate highway with millions of cars and trucks speeding by every day. Millions. The point? One starts looking at his life, his present and his past, and wonders what's still left for him in the future. He was never able to do all that he wanted—or the way he wanted—and now, the rest of his life is good for what exactly? Does he write an autobiography, like president's do—that few will read—build a scale model airplane to fly and crash ceremoniously, dig a big hole for a new septic tank, or paint his house one last time? "What's the use," he asks himself, "let it rot; I'll be gone soon. Someone else can deal with it." His children are always coming by for a handout, they may even want to move in…oh Hell no! He finds he must work at his career longer, to at least age seventy—and longer—to pay the bills. One used to be able to retire at fifty-five even when his salary was the sole income of the entire family! Then, when you're finally retired, your hopes for travel are dashed do to health problems, family issues, or prey tell, old frickin' age.

I no longer—if I ever did—want to go to anyone's funeral, especially my own. As one approaches the ripe-old age of 70, the funerals of my family and friends become a real common nuisance. In fact, I have decided to just skip my own funeral, I mean, I have put out the word that I don't want a funeral of any kind, and my significant other should tell those interested that I decided to go on a nice long trip with no plans to return. I also want to be cremated instead of buried six-feet under, sooooooo much cheaper—and easier to execute—though one does not obtain much combustible material for the fireplace.

I look at the world differently now. It seems strange and new, fresh somehow. As I mentioned earlier, environmental odors are much more intense. Smells intensified—blooming plants, tree bark, people cooking in their homes, the smell of creosote on a power pole! Maybe it's just that my sinuses are clear for a change. How wonderful, but then I walk past a *Dempsty Dumpster* trash bin and wish I had some serious sinus congestion.

In the early-morning light, there's an unreality to my environment—the long shadows, glistening green back-lit carpet grass… maybe I'm already dead and this is another world…hopefully.

All the people you know and love, people you came to know over these many years—there's no time to keep up with them all. Hundreds of email contacts on my computer—literally thousands of former friends (maybe even some fellow inmates)—and an address book so thick that pages are falling out on the floor and ending up in the kitchen's trashcan. You feel guilty for not staying in touch with every last one of the friends you once knew. Maybe I could do an impersonal mass mailing to them all? Better than nothing, right?

Well, I'm not ready for this declining phase of my life. I may just skip it altogether, ignoring this eventuality by just staying occupied. I still think that "you are only as old as you feel," and I don't feel old yet even though this new world around me makes me want to be. I solve the problem by not looking in the mirror. I solve the problem by walking at least three mile a day. I solve the problem by staying busy.

I can only hope this depressed, hopeless state is just a period of transition, with a new, fun, exciting world soon to present itself.

So lets get with it, moving forward…until we drop dead.

—Don Kirk, Dec 2016, 2022

There is some hope. Getting old is like riding a bicycle up a steep hill, there is eventually a good, swift, exciting, downside.

Suicide Is Painless
A Solution To Living
—By Jason D. Potts, 2017

(PLEASE NOTE: Nothing in this story condones committing suicide. It is intended for entertainment purposes only.)

Enough already!

I, Jason Potts, age 64, balding and burdened with a bad back, was tired of the junk mail crammed into my large, rusted, black rural mailbox (a long row of them at my apartment complex—a former highway motel). I'd have to go through oodles of worthless ads to find the important mail, like the equally unwanted IRS statements and county tax bills. I went to the post office and they said they couldn't stop the advertising brochures; it was important income for them. Using land-transmitted mail was down as it was—headed for collapse like the 1800's *Pony Express*—so I had an idea. I drilled a one-inch hole in the back of my mailbox and waited. This was early summer, and it wasn't long before some red wasps had built a good-sized nest inside the mailbox. Not long after that, the mailman, for some reason, quit delivering my mail. Mission accomplished, though I had hoped it would have been the much-more painful and skin-swelling yellow jackets. I don't know if a mailman can sue for yellow jacket injuries.

Then I contacted the post office to get my mail transferred elsewhere. I filled out the required self-addressed card and mailed it. I didn't want to provide a forwarding address, but the post office required it, so I wrote in an address for Candelaria, Texas, a small town of less than 50 inhabitants on the Mexican border west of *Big Bend* in the desolate, hard rock and dry sand of the *Chihuahuan Desert*. A walk through the entire town would take less than two minutes and you'd most likely see only a dog or two and they'd ignore you, having their noses focused on the ground looking for food scraps. I expected, I had hoped, for my mail to get lost there. I figured I'd be able to deal with the IRS and county taxes online.

But my *Microsoft Surface Pro* laptop computer was also getting bombarded with junk emails from all manner of sources. Our government had done nothing to outlaw this practice, though they had been conferencing about junk emails and listening to the many complaints from the public. For sure, I needed to cancel my current email account and set up a new one…or none at all. Real peace is having no phone ringing and no email deliveries.

The next thing I had to do was move out of my small rent house in New Braunfels, Texas in order to "disappear." I held a weekend "estate" sale, sold my 1985 refrigerator, a worn-out 1950's laminated kitchen table, my grandmother's cutlery, a bookshelf filled with books no one will ever read and sundry other junk. Finally, everything sold, feeling unencumbered, I made a beeline down IH35 in my 1976 station wagon to a nearby city: Von Ormy just south of San Antonio, Texas.

With the proceeds from the estate sale, I moved into a beat-up, faded O.D. green, metal-clad 1950's *Pacemaker* travel trailer that was tied to the ground in a trailer park in Von Ormy. I made damn sure not to have any mail forwarded there—I had *Candelaria*. The battered travel trailer came furnished with a large box fan, a *Radio Shack* television, a raggedy old, putrid green, woven-cloth couch, a few clothes with house paint splotches on them, and a well-worn *Sears* mattress lying "flat" on a sagging floor. Watching disgusting black-winged cockroaches scurry about was a small price to pay for freedom. I was, finally, in a new city with no connections to my past—hurrah, hurray!

I sat quietly in my new digs watching a movie on my prized laptop; a wonderment made possible by the brilliant Bill Gates. I used the laptop for some business work building websites for small businesses, but became thoroughly exhausted with that activity. I had needed just enough money to pay for the trailer-house rent and some grub; *MacDonald's* 2-for-1 cheeseburgers would have to do. I had quietly lost weight and so required very little sustenance to stay conscious. I no longer talked to any former friends, what few there were in the first place. I had virtually no furniture, just what was already in the trailer and what I brought from the apartment: a small table to sit at with my laptop, a twin bed, frying pan, toaster, a small box refrigerator, my video camera, and just one drinking glass, plate, fork, knife, and soup spoon. That's all I required; I wasn't expecting, or desirous of company. I had no family left; my parents had all died and I never married or had children. Life was rather peaceful for me: no family problems, a plugged-up sink drain now and then, or a power outage from not paying the bill. After that, I lost my *Radio Shack* retail service job and was beginning to wonder why I should carry on? One day the toilet stopped cutting off after a refill, the sink drain backed up, the A.C. window unit quit running, and the 60-watt bare light bulb dangling from the living room ceiing, decided not to come on. I know it's the job of my landlord, but just try to get hold of him. Enough already. To top it all off, I saw the mailman cramming more junk mail into my frickin' mailbox!

I quit going to my scheduled bi-annual trips to the dentist and threw away the last of my dental floss. I cancelled my annual visit to my doctor and stopped taking the prescription drugs prescribed by him for high blood pressure and for various food and airborne allergies. I felt empowered! I knew an old lady—now ninety-nine years of age—who never went to the doctor even when giving birth to two children, so why should I take pills and see some medical practitioner?

The world around me was becoming an illusion, not quite a reality anymore. I looked out the windshield of my car and watched thousands of cars zipping by at over seventy-miles per hour. Was I watching today's living world or illusionary celluloid? I looked at everything—television programming, pretty faces, and massive airplanes with hundreds of passengers taking off every few minutes—and saw the daily grind of routine, regimen, and rigmarole, and still so much more of the same. Rows, rows, and more rows of identical apartments with miles, miles, and more miles of front doors and only one window to the outside. All I could see was a beehive of busy brainless bees. They always seemed to be working, but what where they actually accomplishing? Honey for the sweet-toothed humans? And everywhere, monster SUV's in big-store parking lots as far as the eye could see, and large semi-trucks moving goods—zillions of products with little intrinsic value—and I've come to realize we're just animals and nothing more, just a large herd of wandering bison going nowhere in particular. It's clear: I'm a tiny, insignificant fragment of a busy, oppressive society that's a total sham. The artificiality of it all! Life's tedious shtick is from the systematic nature of it all. We get up in the morning and go to bed at night, 365 days, and sometimes more, a year. We find humans fighting among themselves as they try to annihilate each other, and for what? I took a stroll in the quiet of night only to see young people talking on glaring smartphones, oblivious of the world around them. Instead, I saw a wondrous, beautiful, glowing-bright, yellow moon. I saw the billowing gray-and-white clouds, and twinkling stars frenetically trying to get our attention. And I saw captivating constellations with, I'm sure, many habitable planets supporting some kind of captivating existence there, but not here. Life for me had lost all discernable meaning; just being alive was no longer enough. Nature is beautiful and all that, but for what purpose? I'm one organism among millions, ready to be eaten by some other voracious creature. My loss is no loss. A tiny cockroach among billions.

I had apparently reached the limit of my tolerance for living. Why, indeed, should I go on? One problem after another in my useless life cropped up. I was fed up and fit to be tied. I was always tired—nothing to look forward to—so why bother even getting out of bed? That required so much effort: making a stumbling trip to the bathroom, getting dressed in my unwashed clothing, and putting on my worn-out laceless tennis shoes. Of course, I'd have to eat something to restore the energy lost from getting out of bed—and that required money I didn't have.

Exhausted with even thinking about my plight, I set out to solve my nightmare. I hoped to come up with several different plans for committing suicide. Yes, suicide, offing myself. Some possibilities would look like accidents, some like suicides, and some might be more fun than others to execute, but of paramount importance, none must do harm to anyone else. No speeding across a median into oncoming traffic, no! No driving through a department store window. No. No knifing myself on a sidewalk in front of appalled pedestrians. Uppermost in my mind, my discomfort had to be minimal because my pain threshold was lower than a three-year-old at the family dentist.

So far, these are the best options I was able to come up with:

Fall Off A Hotel Balcony. I would search out a high-rise hotel in downtown San Antonio that had an outdoor balcony. The night's rental rate wouldn't be cheap, but the view, maybe of the River-walk, would be great. That night I would be able to see rows and rows of open hotel-room windows across the street. That would beat a West Texas Motel 6 any day of the week and would likely be more fun for the forensic experts of the Crime Scene Unit. A balcony with access, that's what I would need. Sufficient information about this can be gathered by phone: an open balcony, sufficient story height, would breakfast be served—my last meal—in the room? What should I take with me on this long dramatic trip…I mean dramatic "fall?" Could I use my Sony video camera? Would it shoot video on the way down? Awesome idea! No chance of camera survival, that's for sure, but it's a digital camera; the chip would surely survive the wild, tumbling trip downward. Forensics: enjoy! National Media enjoy!

Drive Of A Cliff. In this option, I would want to do it in Colorado where I know many of the mountain roads have no roadside barriers. There are no guardrails or bollards with steel cables and no large boulders to hinder my way. On one of the high-mountain roads in Colorado—I have one in mind a few miles north of Cañon City that I've already reconnoitered—I can easily drive off the cliff for a long fall that would surely destroy the vehicle and kill me almost instantly. Almost instantly.

Death by Train. This would require that I walk a mile or two to the nearest active railroad right-of-way. I'm lucky to have a rail line passing near my travel trailer that carries frequent freight trains so my waiting time would be short. I would dress in T-shirt and hiking shorts with no billfold or identification on me. I would have already picked a spot in a drainage ditch or under a railway bridge where I could wait quietly for the next train. When I heard the locomotive approaching, I'd climb up on the track bed and lie lengthwise on one of the rails face down with my legs facing toward the oncoming train. My legs would be slightly spread and my arms out to give me support and keep me centered on the rail. That way, nothing, absolutely nothing, of my torso and head would remain—only two legs and two arms for the buzzards to enjoy. Forensics would still be able to identify me using one of my remaining digits; a finger pressed into an inkpad would surely identify me. When I was drafted into the army they took my fingerprints—all ten digits—so identification shouldn't be a problem. I don't know why the army didn't also take my toe prints, sure might have helped if I'd been blown up in a warzone bombing.

Gunshot to the Head. This option would be a bloody mess. Bright red blood splattered all over the furniture, television, and metal walls of my trailer. Harder to resell it. No, I didn't want that, but the Microsoft laptop would actually look awesomely apropos if I had been watching a bloody horror movie when I did the deed! Ah no, better if I found a nice quiet spot in the woods, but then again, wooded areas were disappearing so fast in the county with all the new housing developments spawned by the 25,000 new transplants coming into San Antonio every year. But I'm sorry, this gunshot to the head idea lacked any pizzazz and would be my last option.

Suicide By Cop. This approach would make a big news story and a guaranteed denouement if done right. I would execute this suicide in a city I don't like, a big liberal city that would bring lots of forces to bare and cost them hundreds of thousands of dollars—maybe New York City or Los Angeles. Only a toy pistol would be needed. B-B guns and pellet guns are now made to look identical to the real thing and are available on the Internet. A CO2-driven pistol is available for peanuts at *Academy Surplus*. I wouldn't even need any pellets or BBs. No cop could resist pulling the trigger to shoot me and would probably not be blamed for the kill. It would be no trouble to fake a bank robbery or kidnap a fine American family in their home, or, I might just drive through a stop sign to get attention.

Fein An Illness And Stop Eating. This would require considerable effort...and starvation. One can survive about thirty days without eating, but a few days without water could end my sorrow so much sooner. Collapsing on the sidewalk from dehydration! But some neighborly citizen would pick me up. One's relatives or friends would likely keep calling the EMS, but since I don't have any of note, I could deny their services if they turned up. Friends might try to force feed me and get those liquids down my gullet, but I would be within my legal rights to ignore them. The pain, and I'm afraid there might be some, would be considerably less if I could get hold of some morphine-like painkiller: a strong opioid-like methadone or tramadol. The drug *Codine*, I don't think, would be strong enough for what I want to do. Such painkillers, all readily available on the nearby Mexican border, would make me grin and be happily dazed.

THE HOTEL BALCONY:
After a lot of thought, going over ever option carefully, and considerable soul searching, I wanted to use something simple, straightforward, and blameless to others, so I chose my first option: jumping from a hotel balcony!

I left San Antonio, headed north, and signed into the *Morgan Pellacio*, a forty-story downtown hotel in a cow town with some size: none other than Dallas, Texas. No real hitches so far. I brought cash, but they did ask me for identification: my driver's license, which I had brought—in case the cops stopped me for speeding—but I would flush it down the room's toilet before the big event. Up the long, slow, shiny-brass elevator to the twenty-seventh floor I went. I carried only my large black camera bag with my video camera with its 18-55mm lens and several changes of underwear to make it appear as if I had no intention of doing myself in. I had scheduled the stay while a convention was in town and I had in my pocket a brochure for the event. I even bought a ticket to the state fair. This was going to be easy. I took my key and entered the room, quite nice digs actually. A pretty, flowered comforter, flat-screen color TV, toothpaste, and a tiny plastic bottle of dog shampoo in the shower stall, but I walked directly to the balcony door to confirm that it would open. It did! I'm almost there, just twenty-seven-floors to go, to be splattered neatly on the freshly top-coated asphalt. I should be able to make a very fine blood-red mess but I wanted to make sure I didn't hit someone's car, so I made note of the movement of traffic at the stoplight. What would be the best time for my swan dive? Late tonight or in the early morning after a big breakfast? I'd have eggs sunny-side up. No, make that scrambled with smoked bacon and golden brown waffles covered with maple syrup and juicy strawberries. That way, I could make a big splash and provide a great meal for the detection dogs.

Early the next morning I was dressed and ready to jump, but I couldn't open the balcony door. It was jammed shut or locked. I had been out there earlier, so what was the problem? I called the desk clerk.

"I can't get out on the balcony? It's locked. What gives?"

"I'll send someone right up, sir."

The hotel concierge showed up and went to the balcony door. He immediately noticed the bar lock had fallen back into place. After lifting the latch, he opened the door saying, "Sorry for the inconvenience. You should be able to open it anytime. Can I help you with anything else?"

"Uh, no, thank you. Well, hold on, wait."

"Sir?"

"Is parking allowed on the street below twenty-four hours a day?"

"Yes sir, it is."

"I see that traffic is rather heavy."

"Yes sir, Main Street is always busy, 24 hours a day."

"Oh, I see, well, thank you," I replied, handing the concierge a token of my appreciation, but I was quite discouraged now, parked cars and traffic all the time—even in the early morning. Hell! I couldn't risk hurting another soul or bending a classic Mercedes. I should have chosen a smaller city…but the hotel wouldn't have been nearly as tall. How many stories do I really need to make a clean squash of it—to make a good meaty dinner for the cats and vultures?

I checked out of the hotel at eleven that morning and headed back to San Antonio on Interstate 35. This first suicide plan wasn't going to work.

THE MOUNTAIN CLIFF:

I sulked for a week before deciding to make another attempt at doing myself in, but this would take some time and planning.

But after about two weeks, I was prepared. I could get to Colorado in just under two days. Packed with clothes, some food and my camera so that I looked like I had every intention of returning home healthy as a tomcat living in a city dump. I made it to the flat, wide-open plains of the Texas panhandle and soon crossed into Colorado on Interstate 25. I'll be there soon, I thought, Pueblo will be just up the freeway. I took a rest break in the "Steel City" and turned west on US 50. I headed for Penrose, a small crossroads town that would take me up into the mountains.

I stopped to take a few pictures of old buildings at Penrose and scored my, hopefully, last meal at a small roadside café. I'm here and I'm mentally ready, just another little drive north on 115, but as I backed out of my parking space, a dude in a pickup truck hit me on the right rear. I put my car in "park" and jumped out… damn! A stupid-looking, heavy-set Colorado cowboy climbed out of a beat-up old Ford pickup that looked more like it was from Texas.

"Oh, so sorry, I clearly didn't see you," he said as he removed his wide-brimmed, gray felt cowboy hat wrapped with a snakeskin hatband. Not from Texas?

I rounded the car and took a close look at the damage. It didn't look too bad; more importantly, I could probably still drive my 1996 gray Pontiac Bonneville with its scratched-up, rust-colored body patches because it fit the profile, and the rear fender wasn't quite hitting the tire.

"Give me your name, phone number, and address," I said, "and I'll get back to you. I have a funeral to make."

"So sorry for the wallop," said the Colorado cowboy. "Hey, I sees you're from down Texas way?"

"I am, San Antonio, but I need to get to Denver; I have a wedding to attend."

"A wedding? I thought you said you were going to a…"

"Well, both. It's not my wedding, just a good friend, and the funeral."

"You could save lotsa time by goin' to Pueblo instead of trekking over the mountains to Colorado Springs."

"I, I want to grab a few photos along the way."

"Ah, yes, the scenic route, but it's a steep, winding road just a-waitin' fur you ta miss a hairpin turn and off the mountain you'd go, boom, boom, bam, bang!"

"You don't say."

"And there ain't no place to turn around or pull off the road. Not much traffic either sos if ya gets car trouble well.…"

"Okay. Okay I…"

"This here clunker, you oughta have it checked out first…"

"Yes, yes, I understand, I'll do it. Just give me your phone number and I'll contact you after my insurance company appraises the damage and gives me an estimate for cost of repair."

"I've got this here garage in Pueblo, get it fixed fur a fraction…"

"Good, great, I'll stop by on my return trip down I-25 back from Denver."

"No trouble a-tall, here's my number," the cowboy said as he handed me his grease-stained business card, then got in his truck and drove off.

Finally, rid of the Colorado Cowboy, I headed on up the mountain road.

The scenery was awesome, and most importantly, the highway department had not placed any bollards or steel rails on the tight curves barricading the rocky cliff overlooking the rock-strewn river rapids situated far down below.

After about twenty minutes, I picked up speed, trying to exceed the limits of this winding mountain road. The speed was exhilarating! The road was loose dirt and pea-sized gravel allowing my tires to slide sideways quite effectively. I could imagine the thrill garnered in driving a Baja, California off-road race, but instead, I pointed my vehicle toward an outside curve. This is it I thought, only a minute or less to go and my annoyance with life and impassioned love of junk mail will finally be over. No more politics as usual. No more fake news. No more lies. And as I looked up to see blue skies through the aspens, my Bonneville left the roadway. Whoopeeeee!

My car went over the cliff nicely, falling, falling, falling, but it soon caught on a Colorado aspen, the largest living organism on earth. My car came to a snapping stop...and hung there precariously! I was only slightly banged up; my head bruised a bit, but I was fine. Damn! How long would it be before a passing car saw me? Too long a time I'm afraid; I was completely hidden from that dangerous, tightly curved road above me. Only some gentleman stopping to relieve himself over the side might possibly see me. No, that wouldn't happen; no one would see me. Instead, I'd have to worry about freezing at night and the vultures picking jubilantly on my nose and ears. I must get my ass out of here.

I undid my seatbelt and tried to swing the car to break it loose. The tree creaked and popped. Oh great, I thought, maybe I can shake the car free. If I was watching this scene unfold in a movie, it would be exciting, tense, and downright scary to see the car shaking back and forth with a loud squeaking sound—and the director would provide a close-up of a tree limb cracking and splitting in two, but in my case not a frightening story; it would be a joy for me to hear that tree limb failing to hold my 2,000 pound vehicle. A hawk floated by, probably checking me out as a possible meal. "Just a minute, yours real soon," I cried out to the hawk as I moved across the bench seat to shake the car loose, to swing it off center so that it would tumble on over. Finally, a very big "crack" and the car came free. I was airborne! What a feeling of freedom! But suddenly, my head hit the cab ceiling—or was it the dashboard—and that hurt something fierce; this was not going to be a painless exercise. I grabbed the driver-side door handle just as the car hit another aspen's treetop and began to roll. The car door came open, was torn from its hinges, and then pulled me out with it. I was airborne yet again, but not in the way I had hoped. An aerofoil effect took me SLOWLY toward the ground, swaying quietly back and forth, the salivating hawk following me joyfully down. I watched as my car careened helplessly down the hillside, ripping into so much unrecyclable shrapnel.

I eventually landed into some heavy brush and tree saplings. Dat Burn It, I was still alive! Just don't drink any water, I thought, and a week or less should do me in so that a hungry hawk can feast on a delicious me.

But it was not to be; someone else on the road—probably stopping to take a leak—saw me down below and called 911.

Not long after, I found myself back in San Antonio, back in my modest trailer, but without my favorite—my only—car.

DEATH BY TRAIN:
In my next attempt to off myself, I planned to make use of the railroad track near my mobile home. A half-mile walk would get me there.

I made my way to the rail line, crossing a two-lane road, and walking along the track's crossties to the spot I had previously picked out to do the deed. It was near the bottom of a hill, close to an arroyo with trees and brush on both sides. I wore only a T-shirt and hiking shorts with no identification—no clothing tag that said I bought it from *Ross For Less* or the *Salvation Army*. I lay down on the rail lengthwise, but instantly found the ballast and shiny steel rail to be extremely hot—one-hundred-sixty-plus degrees hot! What now? I realized that I should have started out very early in the morning, but there was not as much rail traffic at this location in the early hours. I could not execute my plan on this day; I'd have to try another cooler day.

The next morning, about 6:30 a.m., I lay myself spread-eagle on a now much-cooler rail. I heard a few crickets and yapping birds, saw a green frog peer up through a hole next to a crosstie—there to check me out—and a spotted-brown lizard that scurried serpentine-like across the ballast. Then, and finally, I heard the loco's horn and a street's crossing gates going down up ahead.

My legs and arms were stretched wide and I placed an ear on a rail as I had done when I was a kid. My life-abbreviating solution was approaching, the hum of the rails intensifying. I grabbed the steel base plates with each hand so I couldn't be pulled off sideways. But quite unexpectedly, I saw, slithering slowly toward me, a snake—a big, vicious-looking one with long, curved fangs. My eyes widened. It was at least three feet in length, tan, with brown patches pattterned like a checkerboard—a harmless Texas Rat Snake maybe—but I wasn't sure. It could certainly be a fanged Copperhead! A good, healthy dose of deadly venom would be an asset about now; the coroner's office might actually conclude this was an accident.

But the snake opened its mouth—big, sharp fangs, with a pink, split tongue—and lunged at me. I couldn't help but pull back and roll off the rail just as the train clamored by. I could see—and feel—the rails moving rhythmically up and down. I could hear the loud, clattering, grinding and squealing of the rail cars as they passed. Over one-hundred of them. I was heartbroken, I was still alive! Having heard the train passing, I knew it hadn't smashed me as flat as a pancake. The snake was gone, damn! Not again, I thought, not another failed attempt at railroad suicide. I viewed the last freight car in the distance as the railroad crossing arms went back up and vehicle traffic resumed, unaware of me lying there in the ballast beside the track. I lay there, disgruntled and disparaged—a contorted face and miserable attitude—thinking how I complained every day about the horrible disheartening world we live in: the politicians, the media, the democrats—and how on the mark those complaints were. If only the Copperhead had bitten me, I'd be so friggin' damn happy.

GUNSHOT TO THE HEAD:
I looked in the paper for a weekend gun show. They were everywhere, almost every weekend. Most of the vendors don't even require a background check from buyers here in San Antonio. This should be easy, I thought. There was, indeed, one the next day on the far west side of town. Wish it was closer but, hey, one can't expect all suicide attempts to be easy. Saturday came and

I took a city bus to the *Texas Gun Show*. Five dollars got me in the door after I stood for forty-five minutes in a long line around a building full of sweating people made up of mostly men, but of all ages, the kids, I'm sure, wanting more than just bee-bee guns.

Inside, table after table—as far as the eye could see—was laid out all manner of pistol, assault rifle, grenade launcher, and even the more innocuous-looking knife. I didn't think I could use a blade to a carotid artery—the blood, the gore, the mental strength required. No, not I. A large caliber pistol would do me in just fine.

I walked the aisles, amazed at the variety of weapons available, old, of historic value, large, long, small, and even the tiny pocket pistol for the lady's purse. A derringer could be handy for emergency protection—but wait, that was not my mission today: I had the goal of offing myself in a clean and simple manner. I continued down the aisles, row by row, looking for the perfect firearm for my one-time use. I wanted it easy to load, easy to arm, and easy to discharge.

What caught my eye was this beautiful Beretta Model 92FS from Italy. Wasn't that the gun Robert Blake used in the television series, "*Baretta*"? Just awesome, what a way to go out! Black, stainless steel, single-action, would fit my hand perfectly, but it was a 9mm, not a whopping .45 caliber…but 9mm should be sufficient for a clean shot to the forehead. And I didn't need one that handsome, but, hell, why not go out in style. If I had been famous, the pistol would bring oodles of money on the open market. Just consider celebrities like John Wilkes Booth, O. J. Simpson, William Burroughs, Robert Blake, Gig Young, and even the Patriot's Aaron Hernandez. Their guns are probably worth many thousands of good wholesome greenbacks! But I wasn't famous, not even known in my own trailer park. Hah! Of course, I remember, that's the way I had wanted it.

"Here, I'll take this behemoth."

"You made a wise choice, sir. This is the most accurate, durable, reliable, semiautomatic handgun on the market. It's the sidearm of our US military and allied forces the world over. Here, you need this nice black leather shoulder holster. You can easily conceal it under your coat."

"A coat, here in South Texas. I don't think so..."

"You can put it in your pants with this waist-belt holster."

"Great, wonderful, how much does this gun weight?"

"Just 34 ounces."

"Two pounds! Okay, okay, I'll take it, no security check required, right?"

"Not here. Five-sixty and it's yours, tax included, and I'll throw in a box of 9mm Lugers."

"What a pretty gun. It's a deal."

"No holster?"

"Won't be needing it...I mean, I'll only be carrying it in my car."

"You'll need a cleaning kit, here's a great..."

"Have one."

"Fine, check or credit card?"

"Cash on the barrelhead," I replied.

The vendor was all smiles. I was also delighted within my very being; I was one step closer. I turned to leave. The vendor called out, "Hey, I've got an original badge, number 609, from the Baretta series, Robert Blake...you know."

"1975 to 1978, yeah, he killed his wife. No thanks."

"You're not planning to..."

"Oh no, absolutely not, besides, I'm not married." I showed him my left hand with no wedding ring.

I returned to my trailer and read through the instruction manual: load here, cock there, pull trigger here, and fire using both hands. Hmm, I'll only have one hand to use. But the recoil, could I keep it on target, on the back of my neck? Just one pull of the trigger, it should be quite easy. I turned off all the lights, turned off the window air conditioner that was running—but not cooling—and unplugged the refrigerator. I didn't want to waste any electricity; it could be a long time before anyone missed me in this off-the-road trailer park. Possibly months! I wouldn't want to leave behind an unpaid electric bill.

I loaded the magazine with nineteen of the 9mm shells. Couldn't be too safe, I mean, in case I missed my target on the first try.

I was ready. I began slowly to raise the Beretta's nine-inch muzzle to the back of my neck. This is it, I thought, my pretty, bright blood will squirt and splatter these walls with a good, primetime detective-show-type wallpaper pattern. CSI will love it...

But just before the pistol reached my head, it went off, jerking violently backward. I was still wide-eyed conscious, but the bullet went through the ceiling above me. The instruction manual had warned, "always keep your finger away from the trigger whenever you do not intend to fire." So much for heeding that advice. I could see a neat round hole in the sheet-metal ceiling. Might it have gone clean through and into a nearby trailer, thin metal and all? Fear rose up in my heart and stomach. Someone might have been next door.

I raced to put the pistol in its box and placed it under the cushion of my green-canvas couch.

It wasn't long before I heard a siren and saw red, flashing lights streak across the paneled walls of the room. I was in deep kimchi now! I'll claim I was cleaning the gun and it accidentally went off...oh no, I didn't buy a gun cleaning kit! Maybe I could say, "Sorry Officer, I forgot to keep my finger off the trigger while loading."

Suddenly, there were boots on the metal steps and a knock at the door. How many times have you read that in a fictional novel? Well, this wasn't fiction; I was in real deep...deep as fresh driven snow, deep as a sewer sump, or a dry, west-Texas water well.

I got up slowly and inched toward the door. A second knock came, this time louder. I unlocked the deadbolt and opened the door. A tall, beefy security guard stood before me. I inhaled deeply and calmly asked, "Can I help you?"

"Yes. Is this lot 3C?"

"Uh, yes, it's on the sign at the driveway."

"The landlord said you haven't paid your security deposit and the first-month's rent."

I took a deep, very deep, breath and exhaled a long sigh of relief. "Uh, I'm trying, sir. I recently lost my job and haven't found a new one yet."

"You have until the end of this month or you'll be evicted. Is that clear?"

"Yes sir, it is," I replied, and asked most concernedly, "Do you know of any government subsidy that could tide me over?"

"Call the city services at 311, maybe they can help you. President Obama put a lot of new benefits in place."

"No doubt. Thank you officer, I so appreciate it."

The security officer turned away and left. I heaved a sigh of relief. I guess my lead shot didn't make it to someone else's trailer. Thank heaven for that. Next week I'm going back to the gun show to sell that Beretta, hell, I should have thought to offer it to the security man; the sale could have paid the rent.

SUICIDE BY COP:

I flipped through a *BUDK* catalog and saw this *Crosman* ".357 Magnum" .177 caliber revolver-like plastic pistol that shoots steel pellets using a CO_2 cartridge. Just $37.49 and it looked so damn real! That's just what I would need to get myself shot and killed by a street cop. It would be so easy. But how best to get their attention? I knew that once they stopped me, all I had to do was refuse to put up my hands and then reach for something, whether I was in my car or just walking the street. So that was the easy part, but make them afraid of me so they'd draw their pistols, how to accomplish that?

I thought about attempting a bank robbery or kidnapping a well-to-do San Antonio family in their own home, like the ones living on the historic King William Street, but that seemed too dangerous, and an out-of-my-control approach to accomplishing a simple suicide.

I considered jaywalking downtown on a Saturday with my ".357 Magnum" pellet pistol in a holster slung over my shoulder; I would walk along the *San Antonio River Walk* to get attention. Tourists with smartphones would call 911. This would be fun. I would take the stairs up to street level. I didn't have an open-carry license which allowed Texas citizens to bear a real weapon, but this was just a plastic toy gun, though admittedly quite potentially dangerous. It was clear, I would have to get shot and killed; or I'd be imprisoned for a period of time just for sporting a CO_2 pistol and acting like I intended to do harm. Too bad I didn't look like an illegal alien. Illegal's are liked around here, cheap labor and all. No, that wouldn't do, I needed another plan.

I received the plastic gun in the mail in two, long, thumb-twiddling days. The Internet was amazing, so was the plan I decided on: I bought an over-the-counter cell phone at *Dollar General* using cash that couldn't be traced back to me. Thirty free minutes included. On the day of the execution of my execution, I called 911 and reported a dilapidated 1991 Ford pickup with license plate number TXS-6382 speeding through stop signs in the small city of Windcrest. Yes, my newly acquired pickup. I had bought the pickup for just $600.00 plus tax, title, and license, and was enjoying the thrill of breaking a law. I threw the cell phone out the window. With my toy ".357 Magnum" sitting in the front passenger seat of my new, very dirty-white pickup, I passed through a couple of stop signs without stopping and made a few hard, fast turns trying to leave some rubber behind. The duty cops in this little town don't typically have much to do and so I assumed they would be sitting around the streets waiting to give out traffic tickets to fund the city government.

I sped through another stop sign onto a street with a 20-mph speed limit, as is posted in most of this little town. No big black police cruiser appeared, so I had to repeat this violation again before a cop car made himself known using blue and red lights flashing wildly left, right, and up and down carnival-like. It could have been the 4th of July. After seeing the lights, and hearing the siren go off, I chose not to stop immediately, and kept driving until I entered a restaurant parking lot and came to a quick stop. The police cruiser pulled up and stopped some distance behind me. Two cops got out, unsnapped their holsters, and the one on my left stood behind my open left-side window and asked me to shut off the engine. I did. And then he approached a bit closer. The other cop stayed to the right rear of my vehicle well back from my pickup; I think he was watching me through my right-side mirror, not just the rear window.

I sat silent for a moment and then asked, "What's wrong officer?"

"You know you missed that STOP sign back there?"

"What? No?"

"Yes, and it wasn't the first according to a call we received."

"I'm sorry Officer," I said, "believe me it was unintentional. I'm not usually in this neighborhood."

"And you were going twenty-five miles per hour. You're in a twenty."

"No! I didn't know…"

The officer took another step forward to look at me straight in the face and said, "No excuse…" But then, abruptly, the officer stepped back, shouted "Gun!" and raised his pistol, spreading his legs to take a defensive stand. He proclaimed very demandingly, "Show me your hands!"

This was what I was hoping for, but a huge, black, square slide, ominous front sight with big round muzzle stared me in the face: a *Glock* .44 Magnum. (I got my gun knowhow from internet videos; everything one needs to know to buy a weapon and do some killing.) Suddenly, his eyes looked past me hard, real hard. I was terrified! I realized he would have seen my plastic pistol in the right seat and was taking a second look.

I stared at his gun and imagined a big bright muzzle flash and a lead bullet racing toward me, but his was not exactly what I had in mind. I didn't think I could lean over to reach the pistol and he might not get a clean shot—no successful suicide there. I figured I had no option but to hold my hands out the window…so I did. "Oh, sorry officer, you saw my gun, it's not real; it's a toy, just a toy! Sorry I didn't…"

"Get out of your truck now…slowly."

"Yes sir." This was much too intense for me. My heart beat rapidly as it attempted to exit my chest through the rib cage. Facing scared cops with loaded weapons was not what I had envisioned. I expected a quick take down. Me, quickly, down, and forever out.

I exited the vehicle very carefully with hands up and saw the second cop pointing his gun at me. I wanted to end my life here and now, but…

The first cop reached into the cab and retrieved my ".357 Magnum" pellet gun. He removed the little, round six-gun like pellet magazine and saw that it had no "bullets."

"Where were you headed with this 'toy' of yours?" he asked, his face not yet returning to its natural color.

"I, I just thought it was cool looking…"

"Let me see some ID…slowly now."

"I don't have any weapons, no harm intended, no sir!"

I saw that the cops were starting to relax, but not quite ready to stand down. At this point, I didn't know whether to just run and hope for the best: a good clean shot to my back; but he might decide to go for my legs or buttocks—what pain that would be— so I followed his order and slowly pulled my billfold out of my back pocket. I didn't want to just be injured and survive. I had, sadly, missed the opportunity for my demise.

The cop looked at my ID and read my last name, "Potts." They had already used my temporary cardboard license plate to iden- tify the owner and it matched my ID.

"You're okay, no outstanding warrants, but I'll have to cite you for reckless driving, running a stop sign, and driving over the speed limit of twenty miles per hour."

"Uh, thank you officer, I'm guilty, I'm sorry."

"You can protest it."

The cop handed me the ticket, then handed my pellet pistol back to me. "You better be careful with that thing. It looks much too real. We could have shot you in a blink of an eye."

"I had hoped…I mean I understand, thank you sir, thank you for your service. Be careful out there, lots of shootings going on," I replied as I climbed back into my truck and eased back onto the road. I left Windcrest as quickly as I could—at 20mph, a prison sentence was not what I was looking for.

FEIGN AN ILLNESS AND STOP EATING:

I lay in my hot trailer, box fan blowing on me, and eating one, hopefully last, peanut butter & jelly sandwich. When someone stopped by, and there were very few, I told him I was feeling sick, that I had an allergy or an aggravating cold. I would feign a cough a few times and snort as if my nose was full of nasty yellow mucus. The curios visitor would quickly leave.

This method of killing myself would be tedious and overlong, but after my last attempt with cops, this had to be less hair-raising. It could take as much as a month if I ate anything, but in theory, if I didn't drink any fluids I should last for only a few days, no more than a week. Dehydration, I thought, would work every time. *Hospice* used it all the time in assisted living homes when a person's future looked bleak—such as a heart attack or unmanageable pain—if a doctor approved it. I knew I wanted to die now and not at some later time or event. My death certificate would probably say I died of a terminal illness and not suicide, though that didn't matter much to me. If anyone asked, I could say I was just trying to lose weight by giving up food...and water. Hah!

After a couple of days, my mouth was drying out and my lips were cracking unmercifully so I sucked on ice chips and drank a few swallows of diet soda from time to time to "wet my whistle." I managed to stay away from any real use of liquids. I would get very hungry around mealtime, but after a half-hour or so, the stomach growling would go away. When my body realized no food was in the offing, it began to use fat cells to survive—after just a few days—and that's what I wanted. What a way to loose weight! Luckily, I didn't have any family members to try to get me to eat or drink or call an ambulance. I just had to gut it out... no pun intended.

Each morning I would think seriously about what I was doing and I thought about my other attempts at suicide that were much more interesting and entertaining than this dehydration gig: I had tried a fall from a hotel balcony, a ride over a mountain cliff, a smashing death by train, a self-inflicted wound to the head, and suicide by cop, and none of them had worked. I felt this was my last hope so I fought to stay on this flavorless don't eat don't drink diet. Probably the *Department Of Health And Human Services;* they wouldn't even recommend this plan.

My desire for food and even water was waning after a few days; I felt quite calm and peaceful. I needed only to sleep to pass the time. To do that, from time to time, I downed a few sleeping pills.

On day four, I expelled gas exceptionally loud and frequently. I hadn't eaten in days, so what gives? I wondered, could the remaining food in my bowels be deteriorating and turning into gas? I should have begun this exit strategy by eating a few bowls of cereal covered with raisins and bananas to loosen myself up and expel all this grungy old food trapped in my intestine.

This method of demise was turning out not to be fun and I began to think this was not such a good approach, though it might have been easier with help, but who would assist: a Catholic Cardinal?

On the fifth day, I was a mite dazed—not thinking clearly at all—when I heard a roar and smelled smoke. White smoke was wafting and billowing along the floor. I looked out the window and saw flashes of orange flame. There, a grass fire out of control, burning wildly; there hadn't been any rain in months. The trailer park was engulfed in hot, crackling flames! Well, that's one way to go, I thought, but it will hurt something terrible—to be burned like barbecue with blistered and peeling skin. No one could blame me now, but as painful as a twisted football-player's knee, wow, no way! I tried to get out of bed, but couldn't. I lay back down and put a pillowcase over my mouth to stop inhaling the smoke and stop coughing. Now I WAS sick. Yellow-orange flames danced on the paneled walls. No more evening news, no more returning shopping carts at *Walmart*. No more working a *Subway* line with plastic gloves, cutting glass for shelves and mirrors all day long, laying asphalt shingles on a roof in the heat of summer, or driving a loud, banging dump truck year after frickin' year. I was free! Suddenly, a loud bang and the front door slammed open and two fully outfitted firefighters entered. They grabbed me by the shoulders and pulled me from the trailer. At that point, I must have fallen unconscious because I don't recall what happened next...

I opened my eyes and saw a dropped ceiling with white perforated tiles and cables hanging on an aluminum post in front of me. I was coming to and found I was in a hospital bed with bandages on my arms and forehead. I was still alive.

Still alive!

This latest attempt to kill myself had finally worn me out... and left me with a few painful second-and-third-degree burns. I was starting to feel like it would be far more restful, healthy, and enjoyable to just stay alive. This attempt at suicide, as legal as it might be, wasn't what it was cracked up to be. Too few people get this many second chances to live. Maybe I was meant to stay around, that I might actually have a purpose in life. Maybe, it was so I could win the multi-million-dollar *Texas Lotto*—wouldn't that be great—or find a really pretty girl to love me for life. What could I do, how might I help those around me, I didn't know, but I decided to take a positive attitude and stop complaining about everything. I decided I shouldn't get upset by the crazy world I lived in, that I should smile just a little bit more, and simply choose to be happy. Go out and have a little fun; read the junk mail, yeah right, no way! The first thing I did was scribble down these experiments with suicide so they could be published in a book hoping others could learn from them.

I, Jason D. Potts, had been bored nearly to death with my life before my quest for something better, even if that was carnivorous earthworms crawling into my ears. I had come to abhor everything going on around me: the cutthroat politics, devious marketing techniques, the heartless government of ours, and the kowtowing to self-centered politicians; but killing myself turned out to be no fun attol. —THE END

(Jason Potts in June of 2017. He said he wanted to tell the world what he had learned, that it wasn't worth spending time and money to try to commit suicide...and Jason, to this day, is still with us. He appears to be happy. He's running a pornography business on the web and making money hand over fist.)

GETTING OLD
QUOTATIONS
From Some Well Knowns

A few more "Getting Old" quotes by famous people:

"It's paradoxical, that the idea of living a long life appeals to everyone, but the idea of getting old doesn't appeal to anyone." —Andy Rooney

"As you get older three things happen. The first is your memory goes, and then I can't remember the other two." —Sir Norman Wisdom

"A man is getting old when he walks around a puddle instead of through it." —R. C. Ferguson

"My mother always used to say, 'The older you get, the better you get, unless you're a banana'." —Betty White

"When your friends begin to flatter you on how young you look, it's a sure sign you're getting old." —Mark Twain

"You know you're getting old when all the names in your black book have M. D. after them." —Harrison Ford

"Do not regret growing older. It is a privilege denied to many." —Unknown

Mark Twain once said, "Age is an issue of mind over matter. If you don't mind, it doesn't matter."

"One of the good things about getting older is that you find you're more interesting than most of the people you meet." —Lee Marvin

"You don't stop laughing when you grow old, you grow old when you stop laughing." —George Bernard Shaw

"Don't let aging get you down. It's hard to get back up." —Stachel Paige

"Wrinkles should merely indicate where smiles have been." —Mark Twain

Weak Or No Signal
—Josh Heathcraft, 2018

"I didn't sleep much and even when I was dreaming,
I was dreaming that I was awake." Josh.

The air is cool, the sky blackened with low-hanging, dark gray clouds looking like they might break into a rain shower. The rain would be good, but the murky, cheerless sky, and humid air felt dreary. No fun at all.

"Alright, come on, move it. I see this all the time," snapped Wesley Strong, an elderly former businessman driving a pitifully-rusted, dull-red worn out 1990's *Toyota* SUV. "We're sitting at a green light because some jerk up ahead is on his frickin' smart-phone!"

"I know, right? The freeway traffic is ridiculous," added Stony Hill, Wesley's passenger, good friend, and apartment house repair-man. "Traffic is always heavy, bunched together, and moving at dangerously high speeds like packages on an *Amazon* conveyor belt, congestion worse than from a spring nasal allergy."

"Speedsters oblivious to the world weaving in and out, changing lanes, doing at least ten miles over the 70-mph speed limit. The highway accident death rate in the US is in the thousands every year."

"I'm sure."

"Even pedestrian traffic is in a precarious situation," continued Wesley. "Teenagers skateboarding on sidewalks. Headphones blasting music into their ears while inhaling God-knows-what in those fancy E-cigarettes. They're living in their own little fantasy world."

"A pet peeve of mine," added Stony, "is having to step into the street when I'm walking my two dogs because some dimwit ille-gally parked their car across the sidewalk. The neighborhood kids are forced to ride their bikes into the street and a passing car is likely to hit them. Bam! Several kids die this way every year in our city."

"And the city does nothing, even with a law against the blocking of sidewalks!" exclaimed Wesley.

"No wonder the kids stay in their homes these days."

What a screwed-up, convoluted, fractured world!"

"Fractured like our politically-divided country. The left not cooperating with the right. Right not with the left. A pizza with anchovies on one half and jalapeños on the other, no crossovers."

"Can anchovies crawl? A few crossovers maybe?" asked Wesley.

"You want to talk politics?"

"No, no, not now, no political pizza while I'm driving," insisted Wesley.

Before Wesley took a right turn, he tried to look both ways, but his small-rimmed trifocals greatly limited the scope of his view. "As you know, Stony, I just had my seventieth birthday and something feels different, but I can't quite define it. It's not just these pretty locks of gray hair that have changed, no, I find I'm no longer a part of my world. I'm looking at this city from a distance. My surroundings feel strange and are exacerbated by the heavy overcast skies we've been having this spring. I can almost touch these clouds. What does this mean, I wonder? They have an ominous feel to them. Should I 'batten down the hatches' or recline in a deck chair without an umbrella and have a glass of ice tea?"

"Wesley, you're making no sense."

"I look at the morning sun rising slowly through a partly cumulous cloud sky in the east and see frightfully dark storm clouds building to the west. Which will win out? A nice day of happiness or a dark day of sadness? I never know which it'll be when I wake up in the morning. A lack of a plan, or hope for a better day, leaves me confused and despondent. But more often than not, the sky eventually clears, all clouds disappear, and a deep-blue heaven presents itself along with a clean, invigorating fresh-smelling breeze, so, in fact, I still cling to the cliff, not quite ready to let go."

"If you're holding onto hope, why are you always so depressed?

"Me depressed? No, not me!"

"And you go out of your way to let everyone know it."

"There's a weather change on the way. With the unstable air, anything can happen: tornados, fires, floods, hurricanes, or sweet little innocent-looking thunderstorms with ghastly lightening and damaging hail. I figure the human mind is the same way, especially mine, it can change at a moment's notice. If something doesn't feel right to me—the world around me not quite right— then is that a precursor to something—schizophrenic insanity or just mildly obtuse behavior?"

"What ta hell are you talking about, Wesley?"

"Plants bloom, each one in it's own little world, a mind in its own bud making a life for itself until…"

"It's cut down by a lawnmower," added Stony Hill.

"Exactly!"

"You're emotionally depressed, claiming no hope of a positive future?"

"My surroundings feel like a movie set," continued Wesley. It's so fake, a backdrop with a few lights for millions of people who are just tiny ants on this effin' planet."

"You have been acting strange lately and complaining about everything," said the younger Stony.

"I'm just venting. You're my best friend; I know you can handle it. Without a doubt, my fears and failing dreams are all bottled up, wanting to get out. I look at this world as…"

"Stress can affect your psyche, cause high blood pressure, headaches…do you get headaches?"

"Rarely. I feel lightheaded at times. I get a dark, uncanny, dream-like sensation even while half asleep or frickin' fully awake as I walk around the neighborhood. Wooziness comes and goes. Sometimes there are these freaky flashbacks! They seem familiar—as if they happened before—but the events in the dream have never actually occurred…very bizarre!

"You know for sure they aren't based on any actual events in your life?"

"Yeah, most definitely. Something is going on deep within me—a warning of something physical happening. A brain malfunction, dying brain cells maybe."

"You can't sleep at night?" asked Stony."

"No hell no, I'm half asleep, half awake, all blasted night long! I have to make hourly trips to the can, probably because of my age, plus, I can't seem to manage this brain in my skull. I find I'm talking to myself for hours on end. I can't tell what's a real thought and what's a dream."

"The screwy stuff is dreams?"

"There's a merging of the familiar with a dreamscape whenever I go for a walk—even when I'm in a store. At the pharmacy, for example, just picture a room full of tall white shelves loaded with meds in white boxes and attendants buzzing around wearing white lab coats and Halloween masks. Was that real?"

"Maybe if it was October 31st.

"That's not what I mean, a surreal feeling. I'm wide awake, as it were, but what I see of the room appears as if I'm dreaming…"

"I don't get it."

"Not quite real. You'll understand if it ever happens to you."

"You know what gets me?" asked Stony.

"No, what?"

"All the candy shelves at the pharmacy's front entrance. Candy! Can you imagine? Is that healthy? Shouldn't candy require a prescription?"

"The lobbyists in congress? Those frickin'…"

"Hey, Wes, watch the road! You almost hit the back of that braking car! See those tail lights…"

"I got it. I got it!"

"You better have."

"Let's be clear, when I'm dreaming, I'm dreaming that I'm awake."

"So? We all do that."

"Not when you're just walking around the neighborhood…or driving."

"Here Wes, wake up, this is no time for…"

"Just look at all these cars passing by, windows closed, the passengers separated from the outside world. It's like that on some days in the early-morning sunlight, I sense a fakeness to my own world. The long shadows and glistening, green, backlit carpet grass looks pretty, but is it real? Maybe I'm already dead and this here is another world…at least I can hope. I'm not happy with…"

"Easy on the gas pedal, Wes."

"The people—doing their daily routines of coming and going to work, mowing lawns, sleeping in their vans on the street, throwing beer cans and baby diapers out their big black SUV's while texting on their smartphones—that's life."

"All at once?"

"No. Life for me is so mundane," continued Wesley. "I walk through a big-box store, a *Kroger*, *Walmart*, or a discount corner store, and they're all selling the same unneeded crap. America's marvelous mass marketing with hundreds of brands of toothpaste. Toothpaste for God's sake! How many ways can you make it? All you need is baking soda and coconut oil. This is America where more money is actually spent on the packaging than on the product itself."

"Flavors."

"What?"

"Toothpaste! Lots of flavors like the many kinds of candy," added Stoney.

"Candied toothpaste to get people to brush…oh hell!"

"You're clearly on an oral-hygiene rant now. I think you should pull off the freeway. Over there, on the access road, a *Starbucks*. I know you like coffee."

"Okay, okay! I really have no reason to be in such a hurry. Why should I do anything anymore? What's the use? I'll be gone soon anyway."

"You're likely to live another twenty years or more," asserted Stony.

"I can't finish the many projects I have started over the years."

"Here Wes, pull in here."

Wesley turned into the *Starbucks* parking lot and found a space without too much fanfare. Stony unbuckled his seatbelt and climbed hurriedly out of the car.

The two men entered the coffee shop and ordered cappuccinos—one a *Blond Espresso*, the other a *Café Americano* and took a seat in a quiet corner. Unfortunately, the booth had a view of the busy street outside, so Wesley continued venting: "Cars and trucks racing back and forth to work. Miles and miles of fast-food restaurants. Acres of cookie-cutter houses, even the ones costing a half-million or more, bunched together, looking no different than adobe pueblos in New Mexico. Identical houses tightly-packed together with barely any breathing space between them. No yards or views other than the neighbor's bedroom. From the air one sees only miles and miles in every direction of asphalt shingles—one big lunar landscape of desolation."

Stony took a sip of his hot Espresso.

Wesley continued, "A world of power lines—billions of miles of high-voltage lines running along every alley and street of America. Some towers so big they could bring down an alien aircraft. What's our society all about? I now look at things differently, caused by my age perhaps. It's like your dogs, they see things differently than the rest of us."

"They don't actually see much at all, they sniff, see the world with their snout. Maybe I should."

"Frankly, I'm forced to look at countless miles of voluminous advertising on billboards that tear into my very soul. Even promotional emails on my computer seem strange somehow…affecting my brain in a strange new way. I'm simply effin' tired of them."

"I've lost you. I don't get your…"

"National news—all the same, mostly opinion, only there to influence, to advance a Marxist society. City and neighborhood ordnances go out of their damn frickin' way to dramatically limit a landowner's rights, even down to what they can plant in their own frickin' yards!"

"Calm down! What does it matter? You said you're gonna be leaving us soon."

"A total collapse of our political party system, that's what's happening now. Hopefully, very soon, the American people will say they've had enough and turn off their expensive flat-screen television sets showing commercials every few minutes and then throw away their smartphones with the time-consuming *Facebook*, and frankly, they should quit sending income taxes to the frickin' federal government. What would they do if we all quit working?"

"I'm sure they'd…"

"My anger runs high and out of…"

"You're losing all civility," declared Stony.

"Civility! So you're saying I'm loosing my frickin' politeness?"

"I should say so…"

"You don't get it. The atmosphere around me 'feels' different as if something is not quite right. Maybe I'm some kind of a sick puppy. I've been having strange dreams, some in an awake state that makes me physically ill, even dizzy, but lasting for only a moment. My dreams are 'odor' dreams."

"What! Odorific nightmares?"

"Not really nightmares, but I smell something strange. The sensation has occurred before, either in my real life or in a dream. And then, all of a sudden, in the dream, I get the aroma of a fresh bucket of theater popcorn with butter, but it's not the odor one would expect, it's different somehow, a thicker, saturated aroma. Not quite what you would consider normal in a wide-awake situation. The sensory vision comes off as a might freakish; not as it should be. My bedroom ceiling fan is spinning overhead and I can smell the machine oil, yes, the frickin' machine oil, very strong, assailing my olfactory senses. The odor makes me feel ill, very close to throwing up. I feel slightly dizzy. I don't think others have experienced this kind of dream; I haven't before now, but I'm sure having them lately."

"Oil, huh? Some people find the odor of a threatened skunk rather annoying," added Stony.

"And some think skunk aroma is rather pleasant."

"You would, I'm sure."

"Up yours with a…"

"Hockey puck?"

"Or better."

"Fishing pole with hooks?"

"You can't make me laugh today. Not with this gloomy atmosphere."

"Maybe you need to move to South America. Get yourself a little closer to the equator."

"It's not just the dark low-hanging clouds that bring me down, continued Wesley Strong, "I definitely feel an unrelenting sadness, a hopelessness fueled by a sense of failure because it's quickly becoming abundantly clear that there is not much time to finish my life's work. I think I'll just throw in the towel."

"Your towel doesn't have your initials on it?"

"What?"

"You wouldn't want everyone to know who gave up living life so easily?"

"Why not? Look! I'm feeling tired and torpid, just want to go to bed. No enthusiasm for anything and I'm by nature a workaholic. I don't like sitting around, I want to do something, but my love of fixing things is getting old because that activity is never ending. I'd like to jump through some new hoops—or maybe not. Even food is boring to me, even this cappuccino—a feeding tube for me would do just fine."

"Boy, I'm worried about you," said Stony, "you may really be sick with something; this is not like you."

"How well I know. I am sick, but I can't quite identify the ailment. Maybe I've got some kind of weird cancer that's just beginning to present itself.

"You don't have cancer."

"Something sure as hell is happening? I'm listless, lost, and uninspired by everything. And I want my friends to know how depressed I'm feeling. Go figure. But I'm afraid this attitude will turn them off eventually and they won't talk to me ever again."

"Won't happen. Maybe you should see a psychiatrist?"

"How can I get an appointment?"

"Jump up wildly and run around the coffee shop. Maybe jump on a table and do the Charleston? Ah, I know, throw hot coffee on yourself. See, easy."

They both broke into a restrained grin and then got up to get refills.

"Can one drink a lot of coffee and still be allowed to drive?" asked Wesley. "Is it legal, I mean, driving with the jitters?"

"I don't know, but I think I'll walk home..."

Without warning, a piercing, wailing siren drowned out Stony's reply. Frenetic blue and red ambulance lights bounced erratically about the coffee shop bringing an abrupt halt to murmuring customers peacefully savoring their hot cappuccino. Still more flashing lights and pulsing sirens obliterated everyone's chit chat as a fire truck driver following close behind had to brake unexpectedly and blow his horn in consternation. The emergency vehicles were forced to slow down, moving now at a pregnant snail's pace. Only one car made any effort to move out of the way.

"The injured party will be dead before..."

"I know. I know," agreed Stony Hill in a sorrowful tone.

"Enough already," said Wesley as he turned back to his cup of Joe, "I'm tired of this overtaxing environment. Me, you—all of us old farts—our senses here on mother earth seem to be amplified. The physical and visual details are intensified. Here in this busy, bustling city, I have become more aware of my surroundings. I'm swamped with passenger jets flying over every few minutes, freight engineers blasting their horn at railroad crossings, and the endless traffic sounds on major thoroughfares. And beeping crosswalk signals, Christ! Those damn ambulances and police sirens! Dudes who think they're so cool burning rubber on hopped-up motorcycles just to show off their preeminence. And those yapping dogs throughout the neighborhood trapped joylessly in their backyards. They see their owners just once a day when their prison wardens step out of the house to put bland, unappealing, dry dog food in their little doggie bowls."

"A few table scraps would be nice, added Stony."

"Something should be done."

"What?"

"Let them all loose. Open those gates," announced Wesley.

"Ha! Party time! At least they'd keep the neighborhood clear of food scraps and varmints."

"Look out cats!"

"I'm not a fan of cats."

After taking a sip of cappuccino, Wesley continued to vent: "I'm also tired of all the complexities in my life, like the never ending renewal of contracts and runaway inflation. Robocalls at all hours—some interrupt my sleep—and outside in the streets: boom boxes, husbands yelling at their wives, and jalopies without mufflers. Then there's the city-code violators who park in front of fire hydrants, in front of stop signs, or like you said, block sidewalks with their vehicles. I get computer glitches at times when trying to do an online or desktop task. I just want a simpler life like in the old American West."

"Hah! You think the untamed West didn't have its societal problems with racism, notorious outlaws, crooked peddlers, and even pesky ground hogs?" asked Stony mockingly.

"Not like today! They just had to plant and raise their own food. Now we have to go to some huge, quarter-mile-square cinder-block grocery store, pick and choose a few things, and then greatly increase our credit card debt."

"And who knows where that food comes from? Canada? Mexico? Or maybe the Texas Panhandle," added Stony.

"Hell, a lot of our food raised here is sent to China, processed, and sent back to us with melamine added—yea, the stuff used to make plastics!"

"Calm down, Wesley Strong, no need to fret about what you can't change."

"I'm looking at myself and all I see is a frickin' distraught old man."

"Then don't look in the mirror."

"I have to shave once in a while."

"I've got two elderly dogs and they're not depressed, not in the least," said Stony. "A little arthritis makes one of them move a little slower, but he never complains. They both keep on keeping on, and you should too."

"Why? There are oodles of notes on my desktop, and everywhere else in the house. Things I need to do are stuck to my refrigerator, tacked to my office bulletin board and taped around my computer screen. Fix this. Fix that. Call so and so. Do this. Do that. Buy groceries and toilet paper. Check the tires and the oil level in my aging SUV. I don't take care of my car anymore and I don't expect anyone to take care of me. Routine maintenance? To hell with it! Wash it, why? Cleaning out the interior, no need. Just let it—and myself—go to hell! I no longer have time for the chores I've done for fifty plus years. I have a city councilman who doesn't respond to my calls or emails about problems that need to be addressed in my neighborhood like the vehicle-jarring potholes, dangerous uplifted sidewalks, abandoned cars, commercial vehicles parked on the grass in people's front yards, unvaccinated dogs running loose, and what's more, vehicle speed limits in our neighborhood could, and should, be reduced saving a life or two…you name it, a lot needs to be addre…."

"Wesley, I think you've had enough cappuccino. Ease off the caff…"

"Just look at people's jobs: a trash collector driving his big, noisy truck up and down neighborhood streets all day long. Roofers, ditch diggers, sheet rockers, bank tellers, welding-machine operators, all useful jobs, but a life, a career doing this? Twenty years, thirty years, the same damn job? This is life in a 'civilized' society? Cripes!"

"You're fed up…"

"With everything, including all of these crossover vehicles: sedans have merged with SUV's and now most look much the same."

"So?"

"So where's the originality, the uniqueness? No VW Beetles anymore. The only difference in these crossovers is the vehicle's model tacked on the tailgate: the *Altima*, the *Accord*, the *Nitro*."

"You do get a few color choices, a few."

"Plastic full-scale toys ready for a good head on collision," added Wesley. "How about cars badged the *Calamity* or *Ruination*?

"You're being funny now."

"Not in the least, I've had it."

"You should get out of the house, take up a hobby or sport…"

"Sports, hell! Can you imagine the millions watching sports on TV? Watching men at a golf tournament hitting little white balls for hours on end! How lame is that? And a soccer game where a winning score is often just one to nothing. How exhilarating! Most baseball batters are tagged out before ever reaching first base. One needs to bring plenty of reading material while waiting for a frickin' run to home base. I might need Tolstoy's *War and Peace*."

"You're off the deep end, Wes, maybe off your rocker. I can make no sense of your complaints. Is your age maybe a factor to your depression? Is seventy a turning point? Do you think you're on the downside of a rollercoaster with no more hills to climb?"

"I do," replied Wesley. "My head is all awash—clouded over in a cheerless world. I'm here a few years and then I'm gone. My head is swimming. Is there a link between what I'm thinking and how I'm feeling? I'm slipping into darkness. Even when sitting in front of my computer, I get these strange feelings and flashbacks. A certain unreality is apparent. I feel weak. I think my battery is dying with little hope of fully recharging it."

"Some of that is certainly normal for your age, but I know you go for walks and you even managed to put new shingles on your roof recently, by yourself!"

"I had an assistant hauling those heavy, seventy-pound bundles to the roof. Seventy, get it? I've reached the limit to what I can carry at seventy and many other limitations as well. And with my enlarged prostate, I have to go to the bathroom every seventy minutes!"

"Seventy minutes, huh? Well, look at it this way, when you're eighty, you'll get an extra ten minutes of sleep."

"Yeah right, but I'm not frickin' gonna reach eighty."

"Take it easy, Wes…"

"I'm fed up with all the marketing phone calls from Pakistanis and others reading prepared speeches, and the robotic callers that you can cuss at all you want until the line is disconnected. And, how in the hell, do they know my phone number? I sure as hell never gave the number out! And the fake, official-looking emails used to break in and confiscate all my personal data in order to clean out my frickin' bank account!"

At that, a *Starbucks* server came over to our table, "Could you please tone it down a bit, sir? We have a few customers express-ing concern."

"Not to worry, I'm not carrying," replied Wesley.

The server's eyes widened. Stony interjected, "Oh no, he's just kidding; I'll watch him. He's fine. It's just that it's April and the tax man is on him."

"Okay, but if he continues to be rowdy do you see that guard over there?"

Both Stony and Wesley turned around to look.

"Remember, he's watching."

"Sure, sure, no problem."

The server turned away and left.

"Maybe we should leave now," Stony suggested strongly.

"I need another cup."

"I'm glad you're not drinking alcohol."

"Maybe they'll put some in my coffee."

"Not."

Wesley got up and ordered two *Almondmilk Macchiatos* and returned to his seat. "Here, try this."

Stony took the drink, though now more concerned about making a quick exit. But after a sip of the almond milk, he made the mistake of continuing, "Maybe seventy is the magic age of reflection."

"Well, it seems so. I have morbid thoughts about life and death with the end, my end, in sight. Hell, my last days could be so much easier—and shorter—by pulling off a simple little suicide. I think of the many friends and family members that are now gone: my neighbors, college friends, co-workers. Getting old is like having lived under a beautiful deep-blue sky only to see the heavens slowly covered over by ominous, dark-gray clouds."

"Like today?"

"Like today. Heavier, darker, choking off life. Why fight to go on? You see, I don't give a tinker's damn anymore! What has society gained by me being here anyway? Are we all just worker bees in a big-ass mind-numbing hive?"

"I hear you," agreed Stony, "Millions of humans and millions of vehicles. I've got the solution for you: move to the country! Fewer cars, no jets blasting overhead, ozone-free air, happily tweeting birds, and Herefords feeding leisurely on the side of the road..."

"Crossing over the road when you're trying to get somewhere. And how about those foul-smelling chickens crapping pellets, skunks nesting under the house, and roosters crowing every frickin' morning..."

"Chill out, Wesley! Enough already!"

"It's my God-damned ears ringing so frickin' loud! My brain collapsing, forcing my thoughts inward toward the darkest part of my being."

"That's becoming woefully apparent," conceded Stony.

"An icy-cold northerner from the arctic; the sunlight barely filtering through an almost-closed venetian blind. That's what dying feels like."

Dying! So now you're dying?"

"All of the world is the same shade of gray," continued Wesley. "My waning years feel like turbulently undulating Asperatus clouds that never seem to go away. These ominous-looking clouds are differing air masses conflicting with each other like life and impending death."

"I didn't know you were a weatherman."

"Up yours! Every once in a while, the sun's rays pierce this heavy cloud cover, revealing some hope, but little of it."

"A little is better than none."

"That's debatable. I feel like I'm rolling around the inside of a cow's colon."

"Sounds like fun," said Stony.

"Looking at death's door is like watching a television signal crash; just a few pixels at a time breaking up until the whole screen goes black and reads: *Weak Or No Signal*."

Turning abruptly to look out the window, Wesley knocked over his drink, "Damn, frickin' damn!"

"It's okay, they've got it covered," asserted Stony as a *Starbucks* server quickly came over with a rag.

"Here, let me get this," insisted the server, "I'll get you another drink."

"Getting old is all about dying," continued Wesley. "All my friends are dying off. A Vietnam vet, I don't even know his name—who sat on his front porch every day for years waving and saying 'Howdy'—wasn't there last week and he wasn't there again this week. A man who worked happily on VW engines in his garage, his wife died last year and his garage door has been closed ever since. The people I knew that were active in our neighborhood association are dead now or lying dormant in seedy nursing homes."

"You're depressed about others dying?"

"Of course, because I'm getting close. I'll be leaving this earth so very soon."

"It might just be more of the same," said Stony. "You've heard that phrase, 'On Earth as it is in Heaven'? Well, what if it's 'In Heaven as it is on Earth'? Heaven could be just one big shopping mall! Maybe a *Walmart*. Imagine this consumer society extending all the way to the heavens!"

"God forbid!"

"We can hope. Will I be able to take my dogs with me when I go? If the gate to Heaven has a sign that says '*No Dogs Allowed*,' well, I'm turning around; I'm not going without my babies."

"I know you love your dogs. I believe they are people too," added Wesley.

"Well, not people exactly," replied Stony, but they have an intelligence equivalent to a two-and-a-half or three-year-old human child. They deserve to enjoy their time here, even if ours is all frickin' screwed up."

The server returned with another tall foaming cup.

"Thank you," said Stony as Wesley asked, "Can we smoke in heaven?"

"I don't know, but you can bet there'll be plenty of cigars and chewing tobacco at the pharmacy."

"I'm tired," continued Wesley, "I just want to sleep. My battery has drained itself of life's energy. I don't know how many volts I started out with, but what's left is mine until it's my day to die."

"Well! That's the first positive statement I've heard from you all morning."

"Sorry about that, my mistake."

"Having a seventieth birthday is really getting to you."

"I think all men and women reaching seventy start to reflect."

"I'm not there yet," Stony said pointedly, "so please don't take me with you."

"I feel like I'm from another planet and all the people around me here on earth are aliens, walking to and fro, making no eye contact. This world looks and feels strange to me. There is a constant wind, ugly heavy skies, and no sun, see…look out there."

The wind abruptly picked up outside the store, blowing debris against the glass windows.

"Maybe you should sign in to a mental institution? It's nice and quiet there," said Stony.

"Weekly rates?"

"They may be deductable."

"Who's the crazy one here?" asked Wesley.

"You're the one talking of darkened skies, discharged batteries, and massaging of the brain."

"I often reflect on the many movie stars I used to watch who are now gone. And, as I've already said, I think about all my friends and family members who are dead. I ruminate over the quiet, reserved 1950's town I grew up in where I was able to roam the neighborhood safely, but where, today, the small mom-and-pop businesses and the five-and-dimes are now gone."

"I have to agree with you there."

"How primitive are daytime television dramas and the robotic game-show hosts? Series television is cop shows and more cop shows, all boring and mundane. Late night comedy is not comedy at all, just social commentary directed at the young. Pushing Marxism is apparently the way to a better country. When preaching socialism, do they speak of Hitler and Stalin in the public schools?"

"Are you now ready to talk politics?" asked Stoney.

"Save that for tomorrow's breakfast. We might even get some scrambled eggs."

"To go with your scrambled brain?"

"Not funny."

"Maybe in the asylum," added Stony, "they won't have television with its twenty minutes of advertising every hour since the inmates aren't allowed to purchase anything in a nut house. They might actually give you some toothpaste."

"*Crest* I hope. Maybe if I've got my laptop I could get televis... oh, do the cages have internet service?"

"I don't think so…"

"Well, at least there'd be no phone calls from telemarketers. That actually sounds quite nice. I'm for going back to the peaceful fifties."

"Then let me see if I can get you in to see a psychiatrist," declared Stony. "If you're incarcerated in a home, I promise my babies will visit you."

Wesley finished off his cappuccino and proceeded to the bathroom. On his return, Stony asked, "Do you feel better now that you've let it all out?"

"Let what out?"

"Your thoughts and feelings. How about us getting on with today's chores? I agreed to help you fix your cedar fence—hopefully to distract you—some lumber and nails to play with. I know you don't want anyone to get in; you want your solitude. Maybe that's what I'll want when I reach seventy."

The two men, one very distraught—the other maybe heading that way—got up and returned to Wesley's car. Wes started up his SUV and then continued talking as he backed out of the parking space:

"I'm fed up. This is a badly deteriorating society. Comparing our society years ago to today's activities and you see great changes already. Personally, I don't think it's cool with so many people spending five frickin' hours a day on their smartphones totally oblivious to the real world.

"You're not happy with anything going on in this world."

"I'm not."

"The next time we go out for breakfast, no caffeine for you…"

Wesley drove into the street and suddenly, violently, without warning, a semi-truck hit Wesley's car broadside. Their dull-red Toyota flipped and rolled several times. A large purple logo with a yellow star on the side of the truck read "*Walmart.*"

Two lives went dark without fanfare; only the words "*Weak Or No Signal*" were still visible as the "*Mr. Softee*" ice cream jingle played on…until…abruptly…

A loud, beeping bedroom alarm clock kicked itself up a notch and rattled violently. A sleepy-eyed Wesley Strong sat up rapidly, awakened from a deep, dark, depressing sleep, "Damn! Shit! Honey, I'm late for work! My boss is gonna kill me! You got anything for breakfast that I can take with me?"   —THE END

Proverbs Revised
For Us Old Folks
—Buddy Sackett, 2022

They say an apple a day will keep the doctor away, but a shot of whiskey will make him want to stay.

Break a leg; then you won't have to do the job.

Don't cross the bridge until the wet concrete after a rain is dry.

Don't bite the hand that feeds you, it may have Rabies or Covid19.

Laughter is the best medicine unless you just had stomach surgery.

A journey of a thousand miles begins with a single step; a journey to the toilet is made easier with a walker.

Appearances can be deceptive; the long white beard doesn't mean he hasn't tried to shave.

A rolling stone gathers no moss; a rolling old man just falls out of bed.

A stitch in time saves nine, but a few stitches of your underwear will help you keep it up.

Don't bite off more than you can chew, you might not have enough water to wash it down.

You can lead an old man to water, but you can't make him take his medications.

And, "Just remember that one small thought in the morning can change your whole day." —Dalai Lama

Technology Sickness
—Stoody Clodhopper, 2019

"**I**'ve had enough!"

"Of what?"

"Computers, passwords, trying to communicate with anything."

"You mean like when you try to call your doctor, or just about anyone, and you get a very long dissertation on what keys to press. Press 1 to do this, press 2 to go here, press three to donate your first born."

"Do I want to give up my first born? That's ridiculous, he's 35 years old! He's worth too much. I just want to talk to a human being and get this call over quickly. Hello?"

And computers, they were once quite simple. My first computer was a boxy *Radio Shack Model One.* To use it, I had to plug in a cassette player, load a cassette, and then download the entire system software and the document I was working on every time I used it, but, at least that was simple and straightforward...now hell, computers are way too complicated.

And all these many passwords needed to access your websites... complicated ones with upper and lower case text, numbers, and symbols of all kinds. Those damn ampersands, percent signs, and pound signs. Control, alt, escape, shift, option, character...yeah, everyone, even in China, is trying to get your social security and credit card numbers so they can steal every last dime you have in the bank. And "GxR637#223&rr&"..hell, the Chinese can't even figure out these screwball passwords.

The Internet business websites are all now carefully coded access because of security problems...breakdowns everywhere.

So GETTING OLD AND TODAY'S TECHNOLOGY:

Today's hi-tech equipment is way beyond what I want to deal with. At my age, I don't want to learn anything new, and when I have too, it's too complicated a task.

Is this just old age—mine—or am I technology inundated? I seem to be overloaded with the machinery and equipment required to do anything and everything these days. I can't take it. Everything is too involved, Byzantine in its intricate detail, a labyrinth, a jungle of things to learn and get through. My 69-year-old brain is not as complicated as today's convoluted electronic equipment, not the equipment itself, the use of it. Press this button, open this menu, go here, and then there, then here, and then...

Go to a website on the internet and you're bombarded with commercials (many links to other websites) so try to accomplish what YOU want at THEIR website. A small amount of text is spread over several long flowing arduous pages.

One third of television programming is just piles of advertising trash 4-1/2 long minutes each! One third, hell, you can't even keep up with the story, all pacing is gone—how can anyone enjoy it?" And because of the decreasing audience for television, the quality of the programming is falling. It seems *Nexflix* and *YouTube* are the new places to get your movies. And California's Hollywood is loosing their market share. Is anyone going to the movies anymore? The large-screen Smartphone is used all the time by the younger generation to do, and watch, everything.

Automobile dashboards, what a real mess...sitting there trying to drive and push buttons for all your needs: music, radio, rear views, climate control, defrost...my 1970 *Dodge Coronet* with stick shift works just fine!

And trying to do work on my computer has become way too complicated; the thousands of files are harder and harder to find. Multiple files on multiple harddrives...terabytes of data (one million million bytes!) I've created mucho stuff over the last twenty years plus...and their loss would be a major loss of my life's work.

I'm bombarded with technology. Nothing is simple and straightforward anymore, even the washing machine: how many switches and buttons does IT have? Where's the ON and OFF button? My wireless mouse on my brand-new computer quits, no green light, and there is no apparent way to change the batteries. Do I need to get energy from a satellite circling Mars? I can't do anything so I unplug the computer hoping there would be an automatic reconnect but no, on screen, it just reads: "There isn't a wireless mouse or trackpad connected. If one is found it will be connected…" But it's dead as a door nail and won't turn on…so my connection to the outside world, and the work I had to do on the computer, is brought to a standstill.

"The phone ringing all the time, the house phone AND the cell phones. People I don't want to hear from, can't take it anymore."

"Well, just don't answer it…"

"It's still ringing loudly, and I don't have one of those phones that you can read out who's calling you. And I don't click any key, not a one, these same crooks keep calling over and over and over again."

I'm becoming totally dysfunctional, can't connect with this real world anymore, maybe I should tune into this new world INSIDE my brain.

My patience is gone!

Tracfone service, I've had it, the price keeps going up for something I don't need (like minutes, texting, video) so after trying to get hold of a real person at *Tracfone,* I finally cussed a few never-before spoken words and took my six-year-old $12.00 phone, nice designed flip phone designed after *Star Trek's*, (that's why I bought it) and I threw it to the concrete floor as hard as I could. It broke into four pieces. I then, still very upset, took the four pieces and flushed them down the toilet! Did I feel better now? Well, one thing for sure, I won't be getting any more rings from those damn automated telemarketing calls.

I still have managed to NOT invest in a cell phone and so my house computer is my only connection to the outside world where there are websites full of commercials every day and hundreds of unread emails from advertising websites.

Stress caused by passwords, yes, passwords—those long complicated ones—and serial numbers, and numerous questions to identify me, all required on everything. PIN numbers, can't use a dedit card without one. I've had my Debit card hacked several times; a new one is easy to get, but then all automatic purchases are screwed up. Cash is the only way to go now to reduce stress. I think even my coffee pot requires a password...and every use shows up on the internet with multiple websites trying to sell me something, like illustrated coffee mugs...and I've never drank a single cup of coffee!

Getting Old Is Good
—Teri Bridgeunderwater, 2022

The sun is bright, the clouds clearing,
To death we're not at all steering.
Lots to do yet, for that we're gearing,
A longer life we're so cheering.

The good old days, to my own self I amaze,
The sun's rays and beautiful Blue Jays.
We want no coffin with flower bouquets,
No funeral outlay and unhappy days.

Like a cozy night in the city's Hyatt,
There's now a wonderful piece and quiet.
Television at the volume you so desire it,
And no worry about your chosen diet.

From home the hyper-kids are now gone,
More time to buy your likings on Amazon.
Not sitting at work trying to avoid a yawn,
And you can write with your favorite crayon.

Your hair is graying; your head is balding,
And the hot water is so darn scalding.
Your knees a-buckling, your heart a-pulsing,
But life: you're still so dearly a-loving.

There's time to visit family and friends,
Since your life, not yet, so here soon ends.
And time to travel to the west that extends,
And follow the latest societal trends.

You don't have to get up for the day to begin,
You can, on every day, decide to sleep in.
You don't have to shave your pretty chin,
Or listen to your neighbor's 'verberatin' violin.

Your aging is nothing to dearly fear,
But away from it, you should steer.
And to keep us going yet another year:
A nice case of ice-cold craft beer.

So until your long life expires,
Do what your dear heart desires.
You can air your corvette's tires,
And clean your nose with pliers.

So getting old is so much fun to do,
Much better than boiling a pot of stew.
More Monopoly and card games to pursue,
Another day to yell "yahoo."
Another day to yell "yahoooo!"

'Tis all for now.
But don't let getting old get you down. You should have fun
getting old. I had fun writing about it. Keep up with your long-
time friends so you can complain about your aging problems;
you won't then feel so bad. At least try to have fun; you may live
to be one-hundred. And blue skies are preferable to gray skies.

Death, don't take it lightly, it happens every day by the thou-
sands. Unexpectedly. So value your own. Make the best of it.
Enjoy.
—Don Kirk, 2022

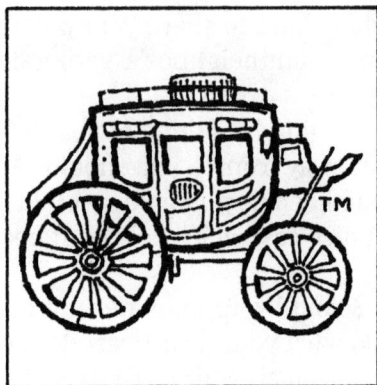

ISBN 979-888796312-9

www.ingramcontent.com/pod-product-compliance
Lightning Source LLC
Chambersburg PA
CBHW062003040426
42447CB00010B/1891